Dr Jean Elmiger is a doctor widely distinguished in both conventional and homoeopathic therapies, and has run his own practice in Lausanne, Switzerland since 1968.

rediscovering
Real Medicine

Dr Jean Elmiger

vega

A catalogue record for this book is available from the British Library.

ISBN 1-843331-90-X
Printed by CPD Wales, Ebbw Vale

A member of the Chrysalis Group plc

Published in 2001 by
Vega
64 Brewery Road
London N7 9NY

Visit our Website at www.chrysalisbooks.co.uk

Contents

To my wife and children
and to all Aquarius's children.

Preface

For several years the patients who honour me with their confidence have asked me to provide a detailed explanation of what they spontaneously recognize as a rather singular and unorthodox medical approach.

Naturally I do my best to outline my methods before commencing a treatment. Unfortunately the brevity of a consultation doesn't allow me to explain the originality of these methods to each patient at length.

This book, written during my free time between January and December 1984, attempts both to fill this gap and to make widely available a credible and reassuring image of the medicine of tomorrow.

I know that any literary act can be deemed pretentious since the writer is always trying to reach the innermost person of each reader, the secret world of his or her thoughts. This audacity nevertheless seems justified when the message transmits a little-known or new truth capable of awakening public interest.

If from time to time an idea has been borrowed from someone else, I have either made this immediately clear in the text or included a mention at the end of the book. The reader is thus left free to find the reference himself, as there is nothing more disagreeable than erudite footnotes at the bottom of each page disrupting the reading flow.

Lastly, to improve clarity I have kept medical terminology to an essential minimum. With the exception of a few easily identifiable neologisms (which I trust the reader will forgive), I have made a point of using only words which can be found in any commonly used dictionary.

FOREWORD TO THE VEGA EDITION

It is sixteen years since the original French edition of Rediscovering Real Medicine was published. A steady and constant readership has ensued, with over twenty thousand copies sold despite the fact that the book got very little media coverage. Word of mouth, always the arbiter of success, has been the motivating force.

The English language is the key that opens the door to world-wide attention, whether we French speakers like it or not. An English edition of my book is thus essential if I am to reach out to a vastly expanded audience. There have been many ups and downs along the way and I would like to express my thanks for the confidence Chrysalis Books and Vega has shown in bringing out this edition.

Good health should be everybody's birthright but alas it is frequently not the case. Somewhere along the way things have obviously gone wrong. And here we arrive at the crux of the matter. The current, dominant school of thought in medicine has little interest in promoting good health. It is, instead, concerned with getting the quickest "cure" possible with antibiotics and anti-inflammatories and avoiding illness by mass vaccination programmes. In a way this is not surprising as its partner, the ultra powerful, wealthy and influential pharmaceutical industry, doesn't see much profit in the promotion of health. In fact, the healthier we become, the less profits it makes! Conversely, the more of us who remain permanently ill – or at best more or less under the weather – the better it is for business.

Have you noticed how there always seems to be just one more river to cross? In the general and medical press throughout the world we are regularly fed stories of "breakthroughs" and "discoveries", which hold "enormous promise". The trouble is we always seem to be on the "threshold", and in the finer print further down the article we learn that currently we are only talking about experiments on mice or rats and that "five years more work will be needed" before the product, "if it lives up to its early promise", will be on the market relieving the by now expectant human sufferers. Where is the end of the line?

AIDS is, of course, a terrible scourge. But it has perhaps one "up" side. Its very name has made many more of us aware of the fact that such a thing as an immune system exists, and that when its defences are breached we are in serious trouble.

As you will discover in reading my book, the therapy I have developed gets to the very root of what constitutes a sturdy immune system and in so doing creates vibrant good health. It does so by removing, one by one, the barriers to this happy state of affairs, barriers created in our subtle, energetic bodies by various destabilising events we have not been able to "process" correctly. One of these, and by no means the least, is vaccination, particularly of very young and thus immature immune systems. The number of vaccinations a baby of six months has already undergone in many "developed" countries is terrifying. But being big business, an industry in itself one might say, it has so penetrated the mentalities and dogma of doctors, and via them the general public, that to call it in to question in any way is nothing short of heresy.

By the very nature of my method, my experience of the down side of vaccination is vast. Of the ten thousand cases in my clinical work over the years I have been practising this method the great majority have experienced for themselves the elimination by the body of the energetic imbroglio caused by vaccination. Let the reader be the judge. Vaccinations are not the only source of trouble. But again details of this await the reader.

A form of medicine worthy of the name should always be seeking and treating causes, not effects. And all holistic practitioners, inside or outside the official school, are doing just this. What is the "underlying cause" that has produced this surface symptom? I have the pretension of thinking that the "sequential homoeopathic therapy" I have developed gets to the underlying causes below the commonly accepted underlying causes!

Finally, I would like to thank my translator and friend, Barry Maybury, an Australian by birth and upbringing who has passed most of his adult life in Europe, notably in France. He has been through the treatment himself and has a thorough knowledge of homoeopathy, so I knew I was in competent hands. I owe him a great debt of gratitude too for his unswerving support along the way.

Dr Jean Elmiger
Lausanne, 2001

PART ONE

HISTORY AND THEORY
The origins of homoeopathic sequential therapy

ONE

Back to school

I was born into a family of doctors in 1935. The superior powers that allowed me this first choice were generous with the environment. The Elmiger family of Lucerne is a curiosity, indeed a case on its own. There are few families in Europe that have given their country so many doctors. With us there seems truly to be in the blood, a sort of hippocratic defect, a vice. We do not number five or six, or even nine or ten doctors like many an old and honourable family, but fathers and sons, uncles, nephews and cousins all tarred with the same brush. The only exception was my father's generation. But this blemish was quickly removed. At the time of my university enrolment, and in the immaturity of my 18 years, I wasn't left in doubt for long. The spiritual head of our clan, my father's older sister (and a woman of strong and authoritarian character) definitively resolved the question for me: I would be the 22nd doctor in the family ... and my brother the 23rd.

I completed my studies in Berne and Lausanne interspersed with practical training elsewhere in Switzerland and in Paris, obtaining my federal medical diploma in 1960 and my doctorate at the University of Berne in 1961. My internships were carried out during 1961–8 in Switzerland and abroad in six large hospitals and university clinics. This classical education and the diplomas that crowned it allowed me to start my own practice in 1968 in Lausanne.

I'm sure you know about 1968 – a year of madness! In France it was the year of debates and student rebellion. For many a dogma it was also the beginning of the end, in more than one way the end of an astrological era, the slow death of Pisces in seemingly interminable twists and turns.

Before the end of this year of upheaval I found that I was also dying, but in my case it was of boredom. After my long and interesting but laborious studies and hospital training, I thought I would at last be able to pursue my calling freely. My illusions quickly vanished. The days seemed endless when spent face to face with my patients: all forever suffering, complaining and resigned. They continuously returned with the same complaints. And yet I was working by the book and not making mistakes.

I was proud of my newly acquired learning and applied it scrupulously in my treatments. But the heart patients still needed my medication, as did those suffering from high blood pressure, rheumatism, epilepsy and asthma. Was I going to spend the rest of my life caring for but never curing them? Despite my deep, indeed 'genetic' involvement with medicine, was I only going to be some kind of good Samaritan for life?

Never! I had a different idea of medicine. I soon realized that I had been deceived. My knowledge didn't allow me to restore health. And yet, open a dictionary and you'll find under 'medicine': 'the art and science of the restoration and preservation of health'. Why then didn't my teachers teach me this art? It was only much later that I realized that they themselves did not really understand the meaning of health. My studies had all been directed by teachers imbued with 'scientific rationalism', reasoning reason, logical thought, the dominance of our left brain. Well, that kind of thinking can only dissect, analyse, weigh and measure. But health is the daughter of life, and life is not measurable. It can't be stopped and looked in the eye or fixed on film or conserved in formaldehyde. It can't be seen, touched, heard, smelled or tasted. It escapes our five senses, those poor lackeys of scientific analysis. Life does not belong to the material world and its compartments. It is by essence one and indivisible, refusing to be split into fractions at the risk of death. What goes on in our universities? Corpses are dissected, observations are made through microscopes, multiple parameters are analysed. Dame Medicine has become a chemist! The primary objective – healing – is ignored.

The proof of this? No Western university has yet established a Chair of Health.

Another element of this deceit was the hospital internship. The young intern is a privileged witness to the most brilliant feats of modern technology. Critical alterations of health, having become clearly visible and painfully material, can be rapidly compensated for with other material interventions. The illusion of healing is perfect, while in fact all that has happened is that a crisis has been overcome. What happens to these miraculously healed patients is rarely known to the hospital doctor. It is the family doctor who takes over and adjusts the succeeding treatment.

In the end every doctor in this situation, which was once mine, is forced to face up to the grim fact: medicine no longer heals. Naturally I am not talking about the minor health problems that periodically afflict us all and disappear with or without medical care. I am speaking here of the truly ill, those who in spite of themselves fill up the general practitioners' and house doctors' waiting rooms throughout the year. No matter what form their chronic illness takes, they just 'don't feel well'.

Believe me, this adds up to a lot of people and is the daily ration of misery that doctors face. It is a heavy cross to bear, and you can't delude yourself for long.

Try, dear colleagues, stopping a diabetic's insulin, or that flush-faced puffing patient's antihypertension drugs or the anti-inflammatory drugs for the gouty rheumatic ... no doctor would be so foolhardy. And so the doctor rapidly resigns himself (or herself, though I will use himself throughout for the sake of brevity) to the modest role of consoling the afflicted, distributing pills and good advice for life. His endless treatments will of course provide relief (if everything goes well) but the doctor will never have the satisfaction of a surgeon who, after setting a broken bone, can say to his patient with enthusiasm and joy: get up and walk!

We are forced to admit it – medicine no longer heals. It only provides splints, crutches, artificial limbs, temporary relief and patching up.

Am I even more severe than Ivan Illich? Do you need more solid arguments to back up this criticism? What would be the use? The evidence is overwhelming! Any one of us can find painful examples of medical failure among family, friends and colleagues: an old aunt crippled with rheumatism despite her pills, a depression that drags on despite powerful drugs taken three times a day, or perhaps some poor soul who dies of cancer despite cobalt treatments and the most modern anti-mitotic drugs.

Medicine no longer heals. I just had to admit it. But what to do? Resign myself like my patients? Join the reassuring group of my fellow doctors and apply the rules of medical school to the letter under the benevolent eye of the great pharmaceutical industry and for the greater pleasure of too many intermediaries? No, the message of 1968 was irresistible, setting me free from sterile orthodoxy. I decided to go back to school. My 15 years of medical study had been but a kindergarten. The time had come to move on to elementary school.

Who were to be my teachers? It is impossible to name them all since they numbered at least five hundred and are now carefully lined up on the shelves of my library (at least those that I liked the most). They are not all renowned or draped in academic titles, but with them I went through three periods that marked my life. I will only mention here the three most important 'pathfinders' of this group.

I discovered the first one in the spring of 1968 in a mountain barn where I had installed my infirmary during military manoeuvres. It was graciously offered to me by the local farmer – a work by Dr Victor Pauchet edited in Paris in 1929. I read it and discovered with amazement all that my education had not taught me about respiratory and dietary hygiene. Above all I learned about that great offender, the intestinal tract, and its role in mental balance as well as in the origins of cancer. The evident role of constipation in breast cancer was a revelation. Well before modern authors, Dr Pauchet pointed out the damage resulting from a fibre-deficient diet. And yet, none of my professors had taught me this simple fact.

Later on I discovered other precursors: Shelton and his school, Geffroy, Carton, Gernez, Colin, Kuhne, Bertholet and many more, not to mention Hippocrates, Christ and even Gandhi – what incredible riches! Even reading the antiquated little newspaper of La Vie Claire (a French organic food retail chain) brought me more real knowledge than 2 or 3 years in the faculty.

This first opening to nutritional energy had a significant impact on my health education, particularly since the application of the treatments I found brought me my first successes.

The second 'pathfinder' was Dr de Sambucy, unearthed in 1970 at the local bookshop, and with whom I discovered the forgotten spinal column, the Tree of Life. I was less deserving in this discovery since my aunt, Ginette Elmiger from Lucerne, was one of the European pioneers in physical therapy. In 1933 she returned from America bringing physical therapy methods with her, and in 1934 introduced Elisabeth Dicke's 'Bindegewebs-massage' from Germany to Switzerland. She had to fight for years against a medical profession irritated by her 'miracles', until finally she was accepted and invited to lecture at the University of Zurich.

Dr de Sambucy's verbose work was a pleasure. His relentless enthusiasm shattered 15 years of academic obscurantism in my mind and removed any remaining hesitations. I decided to use one of the simplest vertebral techniques, Hunecke's 'neural therapy', which I had learned in Germany in 1965. Common sense, however, prevented me from practising manual techniques. This would really have been a second and different profession and one for which I was neither prepared nor well disposed. The later discovery of osteopathy confirmed this feeling, as I then realized that an entire second life would be needed to master it. And so I sought competent hands elsewhere to take care of my patients. They weren't easy to find, but once discovered their results were eloquent. Since then I have acquired boundless admiration for these craftsmen of vertebrate energy.

The third of my 'pathfinders' was Dr J. Ménétrier who introduced me to the fabulous world of ionized energy, the key to biochemistry. I had never heard of his biological catalysis or his diathesis, and you can imagine my indignation at this unforgivable 'oversight' when one of my patients was kind enough to introduce me to his work in 1972. This already old (dating to 1954) and remarkably simple therapeutic method is still not officially taught. I personally wouldn't now know how to work without it, and I highly recommend young doctors to become familiar with his techniques.

The judicious administration of his oligo-elements (*see* Glossary) brought further success and encouraged me in my new therapeutic options. It also had an immediate and stimulating effect on my 'schoolboy' curiosity because the study of catalysis through oligo-elements leads on naturally to that of the diatheses, or, in other words, to the infamous constitutional morbid predispositions of which the old 19th-century clinicians had been so fond. Those forgotten masters, who still knew the merits of observation, found it quite normal that in each generation a tubercular family would produce new tubercular individuals, or that a family of asthmatics or syphilitics could be recognized by the stigma of its descendants. This knowledge still exists in our rural areas, but modern practitioners, having now become excellent chemists, will treat you with disdain should you innocently request that they correct your genetic patrimony, your ancestral energy.

By now you have probably noticed that I have used the word 'energy' three times already. Keep this in mind as you read on because it will continue to appear with growing insistence. It is the Ariadne's thread of a medicine that heals.

The study of predispositions should normally have led me to discover the medical discipline for which it is the major preoccupation: homoeopathy. However, a strong psychological block held me back since my father's health had been seriously impaired by an improperly conducted homoeopathic treatment.

And so, during 1970–3 I completed my primary education, devouring the literature of 'parallel' medicine. Everything that holds even a grain of hope must interest a doctor. I found treasures: aromatherapy, Paracelsus' alchemy and Ayurvedic medicine, as well as that of Tibetan lamas and African witchdoctors. In no particular order I also studied anthroposophic, Chinese and astrological medicine (I'll spare you the hundreds of titles), and am convinced that an initiation into the great esoteric tradition is an indispensable part of a doctor's training. Our science would have progressed by half a century if American universities had studied at the time the prodigious 'readings' of Edgar Cayce.

I've spoken to you of books. Their power is great, but only meetings can truly shape destiny. Mine was shaped by the successive encounters of three men: a pioneer, a researcher and a homoeopathic doctor.

The first was the renowned Dr Niehans, doctor to Pope Pius XII and to Conrad Adenauer, who lived a few kilometres from my home on the shore of Lake Geneva. As a family friend he had very kindly proposed to my father in 1955 that I become his assistant in Rome. This apprenticeship at his pontifical medical academy was obviously not recognized by our university authorities, and I was stupid enough to turn down the wonderful year of golden opportunities being offered. I regret it to this day. Particularly since I would have been living like a prince in the Vatican Palace itself with my cousin Colonel H Pfyffer v Altishofen, the tenth of his name to head the Swiss Guards over the last 3 centuries.

It was not until 16 years later that I was to see the famous doctor again. A noble and elderly man of imposing stature received me in the villa inherited from his relative Kaiser Wilhelm II. He presented the broad lines of his method in the vague jargon of an empiricist and under the silent looks of Pius XII and Wilhelm II. He gave me all his published work, which I read the same evening without finding a satisfying scientific basis. This gifted experimenter had developed a novel method of immunization although lacking any knowledge of modern immunology. But the treatment seemed to me to be somewhat dangerous, and I never used it. The cost was beyond the means of my patients in any event. Yet I was seduced by the idea of stimulating the defence system through an influx of new cells. It represented an enormous therapeutic enrichment and a great hope, a new source of healing energy. But Niehans was neither the first nor the only one working in this direction. One of my patients mentioned a researcher in Lausanne who had developed a similar serum that was easier to work with. Despite the very negative initial opinion of our local medical community, I decided to see him.

He was a Frenchman named Jean Thomas living nearby and purporting to be a doctor. Although not authorized to practise, he discreetly and with apparent impunity saw a large number of patients who were mostly French and had come to the 'source' of a 'miracle medicine' that was forbidden in France. I went to see him and was received in a plain office, which had been set up in his laboratory. He assessed me distrustfully, decided that I was harmless and ended up explaining in a half-hour what little he knew himself of this 'serocytol therapy', which, although he had not invented, he had at least perfected.

This first meeting was enough to convince me that, as with Niehans, he had not mastered immunology. I did, however, grasp the tremendous advantage of his method, which selectively stimulated the immunological defences of each deficient organ or tissue. Many doctors, mostly French homoeopathic doctors, had tried this new therapy and had in fact met at a conference in 1967 to discuss it. Fifty-seven of them had already published the very encouraging results they had obtained. Convinced by their testimony that the 'serums' were harmless, I tested their remarkable properties myself in 1972. I rapidly acquired a solid experience with serocytol therapy through systematic verification in a vast range of illnesses. Three years later I was able to do a presentation on it myself during the fifth conference devoted to the discipline. In addition to the 840 observations presented at that time, 5,000 more have now been added. I have rarely been disappointed by the discerning use of this auxiliary treatment, which is either unknown or unaccepted by the vast majority of my colleagues.

A child likes his first years at school; everything is new, and he enjoys everything, especially the practical work. Thus is his interest aroused and he is then ready to move on to higher classes. The time had come for me to go to high school.

After a while it becomes known in a community when a doctor cures digestive problems using ridiculous suppositories, dietary changes and fasting; treats rheumatism with oligo-elements, cures heart problems through vertebral manipulation and attacks bacteria by organizing biological resistance. This is particularly true when the patients become healthy and when the 90 other internists in town are still using Valium, Tandearil, Voltarene, cortisone and penicillin. My work had therefore become known, and on the morning of 26 April 1975 I received the following letter:

> Dear colleague,
>
> I believe that you are interested in a broader therapeutic approach. For your information, I have very discreetly started a monthly class (Saturday – Sunday) teaching my understanding of the basics of pathogenesis following thirty years of investigation and practice, etc...
>
> Dr Dominique Senn, Lausanne

I didn't know the writer of this letter personally, and in fact had barely even heard of him. He was proposing a meeting for the following Saturday. My pharmacist, who had known Dr Senn for many years, informed me that he was one of the best-known homoeopaths in the country. No high-society doctor could claim to have cared for as many crowned heads as this very democratic Swiss-German. He had been doctor to the Aga Kahn and Shah of Iran and still took care of the members of a ruling family, several important figures of society and many of the most illustrious personalities of international finance and politics. Intrigued by this information I arrived at his door at 18 avenue d'Ouchy on Saturday 3 May 1975. This third encounter was to alter my destiny in a profound way.

TWO

The turning point

I had expected an ageing playboy and was agreeably surprised by the simple greeting and courteous manner of my illustrious colleague. He was recovering from a serious illness that had forced him to stop all activity for a year. I had by chance treated certain of his patients during this period and they had told him of my methods. He thanked me and asked how it had come about that I too had decided to leave the stifling air of the faculty.

As I went through my story, I saw him nodding in approval, smiling in agreement and increasingly amused. He then told me the story of his life, which to my great surprise had taken (more boldly and many years earlier) the same path as my own. He not only knew the methods, but also the men who had invented them. Hunecke? They had worked together in Düsseldorf. Ménétrier? He had known him in Paris and they continued a correspondence. Thomas? He had lodged and helped him get started in Lausanne. He had experimented with all the methods which I so naively believed myself to be alone in practising in our city. Of course there were 20 years of difference in our ages, but I was astounded by this evocation of his career. His story was like a wonderful old movie of which mine was a poor remake.

But Dr Senn had another immense advantage over me. In this race towards health he had a good length's lead on me: he was also a homoeopath. He belonged to that elite which for one hundred and seventy-four years had continued Hahnemann's struggle for the advance of Medicine. I had met a few homoeopaths at conferences, and had appreciated the rare open-mindedness of these colleagues who curiously all spoke of predispositions … and energy. I was only an ordinary doctor, an 'allopath' in their terms, a qualified specialist who had advanced considerably in the art of healing, but who in fact knew only half of his calling. I was really only a half-doctor! Bitterly realizing the extent of this gap, I decided on the spot to learn at last this subtle complement to our art.

Dr Senn kindly offered to become my mentor. This stroke of luck was too great to pass over as it is precisely the absence of a guide that prevents most students from entering the jungle of homoeopathy on their own. (This major discipline is still not taught at university.) I therefore readily accepted his offer, and my high-school education began that morning. I won't summarize here what that first masterly lesson taught me, you will discover that later. Concretely, though, it can be expressed in one succinct sentence: 'Life is nothing but the unfolding of vital energy'.

Samuel Hahnemann, the founder of homoeopathy, had already understood this idea perfectly at the end of the 18th century, as had all great doctors before him. I am speaking here of the truly great, those who cured all illnesses. Yes, they healed, those now half-legendary figures: Paracelsus, the great Swiss doctor and 'miracle worker' of the 16th century, who was even able to cure epilepsy, Hippocrates, 23 centuries before our antibiotics, who cured tuberculosis and cholera, and what miracles must have been accomplished by the immortal Imhotep 43 centuries ago for him to have been named a god? Do you want to know their secret? It is invariably the same over the years: they all flirted with vital energy.

Dr Senn didn't teach me the exact nature of this energy on that Saturday or indeed even later. No one would dare pretend to be able to explain it fully. Later on I will share with you what little I know of it myself. But that morning in the office of my new teacher, the mere reference to it was enough to tear away the cloak of obscurantism in which the faculty had so successfully shrouded my right brain. Everything became clear, instantly.

At last I understood the reason for my modest successes. Since I had 'gone back to school' I had been using, on a daily basis, efficient techniques all of which had one point in common: they stimulated vital energy – do you remember? – dietary energy, vertebral energy, ionization energy. All my methods bore a family resemblance. Even my failures resembled each other like cousins. When the tissues decayed despite the best care, when the organs ceased to function, I had often suspected a flaw of the spinal column, of the bone marrow, as if an electrical current no longer passed. I had been on the verge of grasping the omnipresence of this vital energy, which I unconsciously sensed through the reality of the disturbances it provoked. It only took Senn's reference to it to become overwhelmingly and immediately obvious. During this first lesson I learned that Homoeopathy was an 'energy' medicine like its distant cousin, Traditional Chinese Medicine (TCM). I also learned the Law of Barriers, the little-known reason for the decline of homoeopathy since World War II. Lastly, Dr Senn explained to me his own methods, the key to his success. Although I had just become his student, in one lesson I had grasped the essential.

Afterwards I joined the small group that he had gathered into a sort of school. We were approximately 12 doctors or students from Switzerland, Italy and France. We met in Lausanne, Geneva or abroad and from 1975 to 1977 Senn tested with us the form that his teaching would later take. He formalized it in 1978 as a 3-year cycle of studies open to a circle of interested people. Since he was no longer able to take care of all his patients, he entrusted a certain number of them to his students. As the first of his student-doctors to be practising near by, I felt an obligation to take in a few of them myself. These patients were also to have a decisive impact on my own evolution.

The Senn 'school' grew rapidly and met with a few unfortunate upsets before finding its present judicial form in 1980 as the Cornelius Celsus Foundation. Dr Senn honoured me with the position of Vice-president, and I attempted to thank him through a few small services. That same year, after I finally convinced him to publish a summary of his theories, I found the means to edit his first manuscript, which is used today as the guide to his courses.

But from 1976 onwards I was unable to restrain my critical spirit, or rather what might be termed my odd propensity to discover the rule by the perception of its exceptions. Finding that I was unable to discuss my thoughts freely with my teacher (perhaps owing to a certain incompatibility in our characters), I progressively distanced myself from him and finally left the Foundation in 1983.

Now that I have publicly saluted the man who taught me homoeopathy, I feel free to describe how, beginning in 1977, I started elaborating my own therapeutic system, which I have been verifying daily since 1977 and which is the subject of this book.

But before discussing 'Real Medicine', a brief initiation is indicated into the royal method of homoeopathy which forms its structure. This brief introduction will be completed by my respects to a great innovator, Samuel Hahnemann.

THREE

Homoeopathy

Samuel Hahnemann was born on April 10 1755 in Meissen, Saxony, where his lively intelligence was rapidly noticed by his teachers. Not only was he an observer of rare perceptivity, but he had an exceptional gift for languages. Following completion of his medical studies in Leipzig with a PhD in 1779, Hahnemann settled in Dresden where his renown rapidly grew. His love of the absolute was, however, too great for him to be satisfied by the uncertain therapies of the time. Quickly disgusted by the mercenary aspects of a profession, which didn't correspond to his ideal, he ceased practising and turned to the translation of scientific texts to earn a living.

It was while translating a treatise by the famous Scottish doctor Cullen that one of those strokes of genius so often beneficial to humanity occurred. The many existing books on homoeopathy often recount the story of this discovery in detail. It is indeed very instructive and I must include it, albeit briefly.

In his description of the famous American bark cinchona – the natural source of quinine – Cullen mentioned certain effects that the drug had on digestion. Hahnemann was surprised by the assertion since he had never noticed this reaction among the malaria patients he had treated with the drug. To make sure, he absorbed a healthy dose himself expecting to feel the nausea described by Cullen. To his amazement, instead of the expected symptoms he was taken with a violent fever exactly like that of malaria. Curiously, cinchona's reputation was precisely due to its ability to bring malarial fever down.

This is where the spark was triggered off. Was it possible that a drug that produced morbid symptoms in a healthy individual could cure a person who was ill with those same symptoms?

Hahnemann was in the process of rediscovering the Law of Similarities, which had been well known throughout antiquity but was completely abandoned in the West by all medical schools since Galen (AD 131–210). Hahnemann was of course aware of the work of Hippocrates and knew that certain of the most remarkable recoveries orchestrated by the great Greek doctor were based on this principle. His personal contribution was to codify this Law of Similarities precisely for the first time and to describe its mechanics in detail.

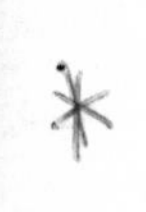

Here again I must summarize. For Hahnemann, as for the great precursors of antiquity, illness is the result of an alteration of vital energy; to use his expression, it is energy which is 'out of tune'. This energetic imbalance is manifested through symptoms and signs, which in a sense form the 'outward aspect' of the illness.

Symptoms are the sensations felt by the patient; signs are the objective marks seen by the doctor. Each illness is thus characterized by its own set of symptoms and signs, its 'symptomatological background'. Drugs themselves also perturb vital energy and are recognized by the organism as poisons. (*Pharmakon* is Greek for 'poison'.) A drug intoxication will therefore also produce a 'portrait', a symptomatological background. Hahnemann, who was also an excellent toxicologist, understood this completely.

By comparing the portraits of intoxications with those of illnesses, Hahnemann understood the degree to which these descriptions corresponded in all their symptoms and signs, with great 'similitude'. For example, a cholera patient characteristically suffers from perspiration, nausea, colic, vomiting and diarrhoea followed by extreme dehydration. Similarly, an intoxication by white hellebore (*Veratrum album*) creates nausea, vomiting, cold perspiration, colic, diarrhoea, prostration, etc., in a healthy person. Another more cheerful example is the sleeplessness brought on by the pleasure and excitement following receipt of good news. A cup of good strong black coffee can also create an agreeable sense of excitement ... and insomnia.

There are numerous examples of this concordance of morbid and toxic effects. It requires only a small step to reach the idea of using one to cure the other. This intellectual process, this jewel of the right brain, is called analogical reasoning. It is a type of thinking that is unfortunately cruelly lacking in many modern scientists. Luckily, however, Hahnemann was able to use both sides of his brain with equal skill and ease, and he knew that the great Hippocrates had cured cholera with hellebore. Convinced that he was rediscovering a fundamental law of the art of healing, he started testing the major drugs used at that period, first on himself and then on volunteers. Using a remarkably rigorous experimental protocol, he meticulously recorded all the reactions occurring in healthy people following repeated ingestion of these 'poisons'. The work led to the establishment of a veritable gallery of 'remedy portraits' which would later form the body of the Materia Medica – the 'dictionary' of homoeopathic remedies. With this theoretical and practical tool now ready, it required further verification, so Hahnemann reopened his medical practice. For each illness he had to find a remedy whose 'portrait' it most closely resembled. The application of this method, starting at the beginning of the 19th century, was a resounding success. At last he was able to heal!

Nevertheless, just as each substance tested on a healthy person doesn't necessarily produce the same symptoms, each prescription (even if correct) doesn't necessarily result in a cure. The patient must be sensitive to the drug. This notion of sensitivity will be taken up later, but it allows us to formulate the Law of Similarity as follows:

> Any substance capable of generating a set of symptoms in a healthy individual will cure the same set of symptoms afflicting a sick individual provided that the individual is sensitive to the substance.

This law is the basis of homoeopathy. The word itself, invented by Hahnemann from the Greek *homoion* (similar) and *pathos* (suffering) summarizes the concept. More commonly the principle is referred to as 'like cures like' or 'pain removes pain'. In contrast, classical medicine (which the master referred to as the 'old school') is called allopathy from the Greek *allos* (other).

And now comes the question inevitably asked by all students: how does it work? Curiously, none of the masters or well-known authors is able to give a satisfactory answer to this question. Each offers a theory based on the scientific concepts of the moment. Chemistry, physics, biochemistry and cybernetics have all been mentioned. The language of computers and physics has also been used, but please be reassured that this is not my language. Since modern interpreters of the doctrine often contradict each other, common sense whispered to me that perhaps the best answer would come from Samuel Hahnemann himself.

With great difficulty I managed to obtain a copy of his famous *Organon of the Art of Healing*, republished in 1975, translated from the sixth German edition by Dr Schmidt of Geneva. This is the masterpiece summarizing Hahnemann's thoughts, which first appeared in 1810. The form is obsolete with its 291 paragraphs of text presented like an old theological treatise. But even today it is impossible to remain indifferent to his words. They have the ring of truth. I had never read anything so intelligent on the art of healing! You can imagine my consternation at discovering such an indispensable part of a doctor's education at the age of 40! I cursed the time I had lost. And sadly, because of 'official' ostracism, nearly all medical students to this day remain unaware that this masterpiece even exists.

As for me, I devoured it! The mechanism I had been seeking quickly became apparent. You can guess that it is summarized by a key word: vital energy, which Hahnemann called 'dynamis' (from the Greek *dunamis*, meaning strength, power). It seemed that I was once again face to face with the theme of vital energy. For Hahnemann, illness with its many symptoms is just the material expression of an alteration of vital energy which is thus 'out of tune'. The nature of this disharmony seems to have escaped the great doctor, who was certainly not aware of the dualism of Chinese energetics. Physics in his day had not yet discovered Taoist thought. But Hahnemann was already able to recognize a purely energetic character in illness. He imagined it as a kind of shock that created a 'disharmony'.

How then to re-establish the harmony? He concluded that only another energetic event of the exactly opposite nature could rebalance the energy thrown out of tune by the first event. Treatment is therefore a substitute shock. This artificial shock must, however, contain three elements in order to heal.

The first element is obviously dictated by the Law of Similarity. It is easy to respect since the doctor has only to look into the 'portrait gallery' of remedies. Let us imagine that one of your children, only yesterday in good health, awakens delirious, with a high fever, swollen face, dilated pupils, and heavy perspiration – a distressing clinical picture. A look in the Materia Medica for a 'portrait' of the most similar remedy (in Latin, the *simillimum*) finds Belladonna. The signs of Belladonna intoxication correspond exactly to the unfortunate picture offered by your sick child. One dose, and in the following hours the situation will have lost all its dramatic intensity.

The second element of the shock is its strength. The disturbance from the substitute shock must erase the disharmony created by the morbid agent. To help us understand this concept of superior strength, Hahnemann used an example taken from astronomy. If you look at Jupiter the planet's light leaves an impression, a trace on your eye. If you immediately thereafter look at the Sun, no trace of the first impression will remain.

Lastly, the beneficial shock must be brief. Obviously, if it lasted too long it would in fact replace the natural illness with one that is unnatural, and therefore harder to cure. (Unfortunately many homoeopaths have not yet understood this!) The liberating shock must be as abrupt as a swift kick given to a recalcitrant machine to get it going again. Another more impressive example is the work of firemen on oil rigs. Everyone has seen the exploits of these courageous men who put out the huge flames of a burning oil rig by exploding TNT nearby. The supercombustion of the explosion immediately destroys the active combustion of the flame. This is exactly how a homoeopathic remedy works. Both the brevity and strength of the healing shock are required to complete the fundamental notion of similarity.

Now you can understand that the only real problem for the therapist is to find a remedy that is more 'powerful' than the agent causing the illness. Hahnemann first found this in the incredibly exaggerated and toxic doses common to his time. Mercury and antimony were not then prescribed only in milligrams as cheerfully dictated by the faculty. He quickly realized, however, that he couldn't continue poisoning his patients, and it occurred to him to try progressively diminishing the toxicity of the doses by diluting the remedies. He thus accidentally discovered that diminishing the dose paradoxically increased its strength. I personally do not believe that this second great discovery (today concretely encompassed in the Law of Infinitesimality) was purely the fruit of chance, but rather the product of Hahnemann's genius nourished by his immense erudition.

You may judge for yourself in the following short summary. The manufacturing process for homoeopathic remedies that is still used today is described in detail in the *Organon.* As an example let us take mercury, a commonly used substance in the 19th century. Taken in large doses, mercury provokes a dangerous intoxication. Hahnemann reduced the toxicity by diluting the initial dose according to a scale of tenths or hundredths. I won't burden you with the technical details of this operation, but you should be aware that the drug doesn't become a homoeopathic remedy until it reaches a certain level of dilution. It is mathematically proven that, once this threshold has been crossed, not a single molecule of the initial substance remains. It is precisely then that the strength is greatest. How is this possible? The phenomenon has still not been clearly explained. This is why homoeopathy continues to be accused of charlatanism by rationalist minds. But the explanation must be sought in the particular method of preparation that the brilliant inventor conceived and called 'dynamization', or 'potentization'.

Hahnemann did more than merely dilute the mother substance. First, the drug is meticulously ground with an inert substance, which is always the same: lactose, or milk sugar. By so doing, in Hahnemann's own words, a 'state of dissociation of matter' is created. This mixture is then diluted in an alcohol solution. But more important than the dilution is the violent succussion that must be imprinted on the mixture with each dilution.

Hahnemann particularly insists on the correct way to shake the mixing tube. The shock must be violent and above all 'elastic'. This is essential. As for the rest, the meticulous manipulations are described with a scientific precision that reminds one of the constraints of a ritual. Was Hahnemann the brilliant chemist also an alchemist? Had he been influenced by the theosophic reflections of his illustrious elder, Emanuel Swedenborg (1688–1772)? This is impossible to know, but I continue to be amazed by the doctrinal unity of all his work in its constant reference to the superior doctrine governing our life: vital energy, or 'dynamis'. His devotion proved worthwhile since it resulted in the solution of the therapist's major problem: how to give 'power' to the remedy? He simply made it 'dynamic', or non-material.

It is the perfect harmony between the immateriality of the remedy and the immateriality of the energetic imbalance, which alone can free the altered vital energy. By diluting the remedy beyond the limits of our material world, Hahnemann raised it to a higher level, the level of higher vibration, which is life.

But let us not jump ahead. You are now aware of the principles of this truly healing medicine, which was to be so successful at the beginning of the 19th century. It is important to underline that, from the moment of its discovery, homoeopathy generated a wave of enthusiasm that quickly conquered Europe and then the United States. There were thousands of disciples and the innumerable successful cures increased its renown. But 'the old school' wouldn't lay down its arms, and its solidly materialist champions were to gain tremendous advantage from the enormous scientific achievement of the century: the discovery of infectious agents and modern chemotherapy.

Homoeopathy's progress was abruptly stopped, going from near-triumph into rapid decline. Once again Galen's spirit, peddled by pragmatic rationalists, offered the easy way out and led to the deadly impasse that we find ourselves in today, ruining our health and our budgets. But chemotherapy was fortunately unable to deal a death blow to homoeopathy. Truth has a way of imposing itself, and is often saved at the last minute by a handful of idealists or even a single individual, an involuntary artisan of destiny. Such a providential man existed and you are about to make his acquaintance.

FOUR

Dr Voll's discovery

If you come down with a cold or a mild case of bronchitis or sinusitis and ask your local pharmacy for a homoeopathic remedy the chances are that you won't be very satisfied with the results. In fact you'll be very lucky if anything like the 'gentle and durable' cure promised by Hahnemann's disciples occurs. Failure is unfortunately more common than success.

I went through this myself while I was still a 'half-doctor' knowing only the allopathic side of my profession. In order to test the mysterious method and to satisfy the requests of my more curious patients, I had made several attempts at curing cystitis or sore throat with certain well-known homoeopathic remedies. The results were a disappointment, and I had concluded (as a good allopath) that homoeopathy was a waste of time. I could easily be excused since use of the proper methods had not been part of my medical training. I acted in good faith as my medical mentors had not taught me the method. But there is a more serious error than that.

This same misfortune has been occurring more and more frequently over the last 40 years, even amongst the most gifted practising homoeopaths. On that Saturday in May 1975 when I started my apprenticeship, Dr Senn showed me his large collection of prescriptions written by some of the most illustrious contemporary homoeopaths. They had been given to Senn by the many patients who had come to him worn out and defeated by the interminable and ineffective homoeopathic treatments of these doctors. I must admit that I too had to laugh at seeing the names of some of the most famous contemporary masters, mostly French, who write scholarly books and pontificate from the platform at medical conferences.

But how was it possible that so many renowned doctors could have made such terrible mistakes? It was through Dr Senn's answer to this question that I finally understood the real reason for the decline of homoeopathy. The concept is best summarized in one word: barriers. With the partial understanding of the underlying mechanism it was to become the key to Senn's success as a doctor and the pivotal point of his teaching.

Where this idea came from, in which period and in what circumstances, I learned only later, and quite accidentally. I got on the right track when fortuitously I discovered in a bookshop some technical documentation on electroacupuncture. As it is in my nature always to go back to the source of information before passing it on, here is the result of my little inquiry.

A new idea generally comes from one person only, the one who first clearly formulates it. If the idea is good, the inventor can become a benefactor. I found such a providential man in Reinhold Voll. But, before I go further, a brief digression is necessary concerning ancient Chinese medical thought, which is the source from which this German country doctor developed his investigations.

What the wise men of ancient China knew about life could be summarized in one phrase: 'Life is nothing else but the unfolding of energy'. Here, once again, we find our old friend. However, what we hadn't as yet picked up in Hahnemann had already been clearly stated by these wise men in China 5,000 years earlier: all energy is essentially bipolar. This is the second principle of traditional energetics and is one that modern physics would not contradict. It comes straight from the *Book of Changes*, the famous *I Ching* of the legendary emperor Fo Hi, which rules all expressions of being.

For the ancient Chinese masters, all expression is movement and obeys the laws of binary propagation, oscillating between two opposite poles. Day follows night, summer follows winter, etc. I will not repeat this archiclassic demonstration; you have of course recognized the great Chinese law of bipolarity which places the Yin and the Yang at the two extreme poles of all movement. Yang represents loftiness, the sky, the outside, fire, expansion, the masculine; Yin represents below, the earth, shelter, water, conservation, the feminine. But deep within Yin there is always a grain of Yang, just as in Yang a beginning of Yin can always be found. This particularity explains the constant swing from one principle to the other, which is the definition of movement.

Vital energy is pure movement. From the moment of fertilization on, it is an irresistible forward motion. Its constant oscillation ensures harmonious growth, structuring the systems and organs. But it doesn't spread haphazardly; it obeys a plan. Like all applied energy, it follows lines of force, the same as those that create and animate our structures. The Chinese very soon learned to identify these lines of force which they named meridians, and the points where they come to the surface, the famous points of acupuncture.

How did they discover these things? All kinds of theories have been advanced to answer this question. Personally, I opt for the simplest; they felt and saw them. With a little training, everyone can become sensitive to the crackling sensation which can be felt as a finger approaches one of these Chinese points. I even know a young woman who is lucky enough to be able to see them.

It doesn't really matter how the meridians were found; what counts is their existence. The Chinese established that this is how vital energy circulates, that its fluctuations can be apprehended directly by our senses and that health can be seen as a harmonious energetic balance. They analysed variations in the vital flow by day and night, seasonally and by the hour. Contrary to what is taught in the West, they noticed that the internal organs are neither separate nor separable but in fact operate in close energetic dependence regulated by connections unimagined by our scholars. A given organ is invigorated at a certain hour by a given aspect of vital energy. But the organ doesn't store energy. Once the amount required to accomplish the task has been taken in, the energetic balance overflows to the other partners in the system. With the skill derived from experience, the practitioner can test the health of each organ and the overall organism merely by studying the variations perceived in the points and the pulses known to the Chinese. An imbalanced organ will be revealed through these windows, showing either an excess, reduction or flaw in the energy of Yin and Yang.

You can easily grasp that treatment can also take place through the same channels. To purge a given organ, the energy that is stagnating on its points must be dispersed. To stimulate another, a supplement of energy will have to be taken from elsewhere and rechannelled. This subtle art of regulation is practised with metal needles or heat. It permits the rebalancing of the energy flow in the whole as well as in the parts. With global balance reinstated, health is guaranteed. The acupuncturist will have done essentially the same thing as the homoeopath. The subtle difference between them is that acupuncture focuses solely on the Yin and Yang aspect of energy in distress, whereas homoeopathy concerns itself solely with global balance.

Dr Voll didn't practise acupuncture, but he knew the principles well. His inventive and curious mind decided that modern technical methods should be able to measure the minute energetic variations felt by the acupuncturist's trained hands. Most energetic changes result in the modification of some physically related and thus measurable area. It could be a thermal change, one in mechanical pressure or permeability or perhaps in electrical or magnetic current. Voll opted for the systematic study of variations in the electrical potential, which he hoped to find on the Chinese points. Experimentation proved him right.

By 1953, and with the help of an engineer, he had built a measuring device inspired by the classical ohmmeter. This machine enabled him to measure the difference in electrical potential between any specific point and the overall surface of the body. It seems that the acupuncture point functions like a mini-accumulator of electrical energy which is more or less charged depending on the condition of the vector meridian or the underlying organ. By incorporating this tiny source of energy into a weak electrical circuit it is possible to measure its charge by measuring the drop in the general resistance of the circuit.

In this way one can obtain a fairly precise idea of the overall health of each organ tested as well as of the body as a whole. Better yet, by charging or discharging the acupuncture points through lightly modulated electrical shocks it is possible to heal the organs that are imbalanced owing to inadequate or excess Yin or Yang energy. This activity corresponds to the invigoration and dispersion practised by the acupuncturist, hence the name electro-acupuncture. The possibilities of the two methods are essentially the same. Electro-acupuncture is merely able to overcome the handicap that training in manual sensitivity imposes on a 'normal' acupuncturist. (We will see later that this seeming advantage is in fact a serious handicap.)

In 1956 Voll started an association to diffuse his method internationally. He was not, however, alone in using modern techniques to detect bioenergetic phenomena. Nor was he the first to use electrical equipment. There were many French and

American precursors of this invention. As early as 1919 a Dr Albert Abrams of San Francisco was reportedly using an 'electric oscillator'. Historical research is, however, of little interest to me. What on the other hand seems to me of capital importance is the chain of ideas that a discovery can set off. Voll's work started a series of discoveries whose path I will briefly trace below.

If one admits that life is movement, and therefore a manifestation of energy, one also has to admit that every chemical reaction observed *in vivo* is also a kind of energy discharge. Therefore, at the beginning of the reaction, each chemical substance has its own energetic potential. Dr Voll began to wonder whether all chemical reactions had a specific potential, the ability to transmit energy – a kind of radiation, so to speak – and whether this phenomenon could not in turn be measured.

The hypothesis was verified by the following finding – that every chemical substance has, in fact, a specific energetic radiation – as all radiesthesists know. It would seem that living matter is sensitive to this. To convince you, an experiment conducted by one of Dr Voll's correspondents, Dr Morell of Ottlingen, will illustrate this point. Morell started with two pipettes of blood samples from the same patient which were destined for measuring the speed of blood sedimentation. Using a special device, he placed one of the pipettes in a larger test-tube containing a common mild chemical solution. The surprising result was that the speed of sedimentation measured after an hour was clearly different between the two samples. What does this experiment show? It shows that each chemical substance has its own energy radiation and is capable of modifying other energetic manifestations such as the sedimentation speed of blood.

It seemed possible to Voll and his colleagues that a chemical substance could modify the electrical resistance of the Chinese acupuncture points. Experimentation proved their hypothesis to be true, and particularly when homoeopathically 'dynamized' or 'potentized' doses were used. This shouldn't surprise us because let us not forget that a homoeopathic remedy is prepared from a basic element and is, by the process of dilution/potentization, lifted on to an immaterial level where life and its mysterious vibratory frequencies reign. They thus confirmed the results obtained by another German precursor, Dr Weihe, who had identified a detailed 'map' of certain points on the surface of the body that were particularly sensitive during homoeopathic experiments.

Voll's team didn't stop their work with these verifications. Just as electroacupuncture would lead to certain treatments, so the indications given by the substances tests would lead to new therapeutic possibilities. A brief example will illustrate the direction they took. Let us take a common case of gastritis. It can easily be detected with an ohmmeter at the points corresponding to the stomach. The appropriate remedy can be found by similarly testing the various chemical or homoeopathic substances that might cure it. This is done quite simply by incorporating the energy of the substance into the electrical circuit of the ohmmeter. There are various ways of doing this, the most common being to have a small bottle containing the substance held by the patient in the same hand as the electrode. If the imbalanced Chinese point regains its electrical balance, then the choice of medication is correct and its administration will correct the 'imbalance', thus bringing about a cure.

Please excuse me, dear reader, if I have bored you with this long parenthesis about Chinese medicine and the ohmmetric technique for diagnosis, but it will help illustrate the originality of Voll's discovery. All of his patients had received nothing but the classical chemical remedies used by 'official' medicine. Some of them, mostly chronically ill, had therefore ingested considerable quantities of these substances, which, over time, had been poorly eliminated from the body. Now what happens when eliminatory organs are overloaded by a chronic abuse of chemical substances (and therefore by definition, toxic)? The residual waste of these chemical substances remains in the body in what are termed 'mesenchymatous tissues'. But these makeshift storage points can also become congested with the resultant osteoarthritis, rheumatism, gout and arteriosclerosis that we refer to as 'diseases of civilization'.

Dr Voll called this common cause of so many ills 'mesenchymblockade'. This blockage of the body's ability to adapt to toxic congestion can be easily diagnosed by the ohmmeter owing to the electric anomalies found at the acupuncture points corresponding to the organs of elimination. The blockage can be removed just as easily as it is diagnosed.

Herein lies Voll's great discovery. He called this treatment 'the reactivation of the mesenchymatous tissues'. What did he do to give back to the blocked functions their capacity to function? He simply treated patients by giving them a homoeopathic potentization-dilution of the substance that was causing the blockage, thus allowing the electrical current to again pass freely.

Homoeopaths call this technique 'isotherapy' (from '*isos*' meaning equal). The remedies used are called isotherapeutics or 'nosodes' (from '*nosos*' meaning illness), and are prepared directly from the toxic drug or infectious agent. It is easy to understand that the shock transmitted will be rigorously identical to the imbalance of the illness. One can no longer speak of homoeopathy here since that method seeks the 'most similar' remedy, the 'simillimum', whereas the nosode could really be called the perfect remedy, the ideal 'simile'. Isotherapy represents the perfect balance between the illness, its cause and its cure. When the isotherapeutic is administered at an appropriate strength, and with some additional stimulation of the detoxifying organs (liver, kidneys, etc) known as 'draining', the organism's energetic balance is quickly re-established.

Voll's extremely elegant method of electrical detection was codified in the late 1950s by his followers. It re-established the little-used method of treatment with nosodes, and above all contributed to the dissemination of the idea of energy blockage, which is truly the cornerstone of modern homoeopathy.

Dr Senn introduced the method in Switzerland in 1960, and, although he never referred to Voll's work in his courses, this theory of blockage became the *Leitmotif* of his practice and teaching. In a very close parallel to the 'mesenchymblockade', Senn proposed an audacious energetic vision based on the hypothetical Chinese law of Koann Fa, 'the Law of Barriers'. This concept was supposedly revealed to him by the study of ancient and little-known Chinese texts. Unfortunately his poor understanding of the Chinese language and lack of initiation into the basic practice of acupuncture allowed only a 'Western', and therefore limited, understanding of these subtle energetic phenomena. This is why the explanation that he thought he had found for the 'Law of Barriers' is essentially a slightly modified version of Voll's theory.

Credit is still due to the Lausanne doctor for his attempts to establish his precursor Voll's original thinking in the homoeopathic world. His first presentation to the International Homoeopathic League went completely unnoticed. It was followed by another at the 1976 congress in Athens, but the presentation was made in an extremely confusing manner and didn't generate any real interest. A last attempt was made during the 1983 congress in Vienna, but was effectively sabotaged by the committee and succumbed under the weight of sarcastic criticism.

Why these setbacks? There had to be a reason why acceptance of this concept of barriers by the medical world was so slow. I believe the answer lies in the interpretation of the Vollien method. Its centrepiece – the ohmmetric test – is not completely reliable and can lead to easy successes that are often followed by bitter disappointments.

FIVE

The technical visualization of illness

A visit to the homoeopathic doctor usually begins when allopathy has abandoned the patient. The homoeopath, who has had the same training as his allopathic colleagues, can begin his investigation with a meticulous physical examination complemented by the usual range of biochemical tests and other investigative techniques. However, this first phase usually proves unnecessary since the patient already knows the medical diagnosis when he decides to seek non-official help. In fact the person is often in possession of a bulky file compiled by the various doctors who have followed each other in vain at the patient's bedside. The homoeopath will restrict himself to the judicious use of this information without however adding to the technical inflation. Since the classic diagnosis is known, his task is to succeed where others have failed. This is when the real work begins.

A first examination, more or less laborious depending on his skill, will permit identification of the 'portrait' of the illness as it appears in the patient. If the doctor belongs to the classic Hahnemann school, he will try to identify, among all the information obtained, the elements allowing prescription of the remedy with the greatest resemblance, the 'simillimum'. Prescription of this remedy should allow the sick organism to find its energetic balance, in other words its health.

Through further discreet examination, the homoeopath will then try to define the 'constitutional type' of his patient. This concept is very important in homoeopathy but completely unknown in allopathy. It will allow the doctor to anticipate the reactional mode of his patient while the illness runs its course. It is not my purpose here to teach homoeopathy, but it is important to know that constitutional remedies are absolutely individualized. They accompany a person for life, allowing a certain revitalization of energy in moments of weakness.

The other major consideration is the definition of predisposition. Classical medicine pretends to be unaware that certain illnesses are always attached to the same predispositions. This is because there is no real choice among available treatments in allopathy. They always remain superficial, whereas the homoeopathic remedy works in depth. (I will discuss diverse hereditary and genetic predispositions at greater length in Part III.)

Lastly, after a judicious questioning or a brief physical examination, the doctor will be able to choose a complementary supporting medicine that is designed to help the organism eliminate toxins accumulated through the patient's lifestyle, diet or previous allopathic treatments.

This is only a brief overview of a homoeopathic medical visit. If all goes well, the doctor will have the great pleasure of seeing the unbelievable efficiency of a correctly chosen homoeopathic remedy. Whether the symptoms are acute or chronic, they can disappear completely with the simillimum.

This was a daily pleasure for Hahnemann and his early followers. In reading works of the last century, one is struck by the prodigious number of near-miraculous cures accomplished with one single remedy given only once. This is the dream of every homoeopath! Today a doctor would be imprudent in the extreme if he claimed the ability to cure definitively an unruly case of asthma with one single dose of Aralia or a neurasthenic with one single dose of Sepia. The 'gentle and durable' cures promised by Hahnemann in 1810 are now operative only for a few months or weeks!

Unfortunately, Hahnemann's days have vanished owing to the universal chemical pollution that is the symbol of our period. But even though today the work of the old homoeopathic masters often leaves us perplexed or incredulous, similar good fortune smiles on each contemporary disciple at least once. In fact it is often due to a feat of this nature that many persevere despite the derision of their colleagues in the difficult apprenticeship of this art.

Every homoeopath delights in telling the story of his first success, and I won't resist this pleasure since it was decisive in its encouragement of my new vocation. I had known Mme

Madeleine Deville for several years and had treated her for occasional minor illnesses. One morning in September 1976 she called me urgently to her bedside where I was confronted by a clear-cut case of acute pyelonephritis with extremely high temperature and significant pain. Laboratory analysis immediately confirmed the gravity of the situation and there was no question that antibiotic treatment was required. Perhaps it was Hahnemann's ghost whispering in my ear, but, faced with my patient's reticence to take antibiotics, I decided to try a homoeopathic treatment. Mme Deville knew that I was taking my first steps in a new direction and her confidence, calm assurance and strong personality helped me to decide. Through questioning and observation I chose the simillimum Arsenicum album. My patient's determined and meticulous temperament as well as her orderly, clean and tastefully decorated apartment, had already suggested this remedy. As a final test, I asked her abruptly: 'Madame, what would you do if from your bedside you noticed that the painting across the room was askew?' Horrified, and with vehement indignation, she immediately replied, 'Doctor, I can assure you that even if it were on my death bed I'd find the strength to get up and straighten it!' It was this extreme perfectionism manifesting itself despite the intensity of the illness that made up my mind. Only an 'Arsenicum' could have answered my question that way. I administered a dose, and decided to check back on her later in the day. I didn't want to wait too long before prescribing the antibiotic which would be indispensable if Arsenicum failed. My academic conscience (not to mention my generally hostile surroundings) would have severely reproached such a professional mistake.

You can't imagine my amazement at seeing a significant improvement that same afternoon! I decided to hold off the antibiotic, and by the next day it was clear that I wouldn't have to administer it at all. The fever had dropped, the lumbar region was more flexible, the pain was gone and the lab results were less pessimistic. Verification the next day at my consulting room confirmed the radical disappearance of the acute illness. And I was to have yet another surprise. The patient informed me that she had recovered her form of the previous summer. I was as intrigued by this assertion as by the suddenness with which such a serious illness had taken hold of such a robust and healthy person. My investigations soon found the connection.

During Mme Deville's vacation in Brittany a month earlier, she had eaten some badly prepared oysters. Although she had been as 'sick as a dog', her strong constitution quickly recovered and she had not even bothered to mention this incident to me when she returned. Well, oysters are wonderful little animals that function something like filters for the seawater in which they live. Amongst other things, seawater contains small quantities of arsenic, which can accumulate in fairly significant quantities in oysters. If the mollusc isn't drained properly or isn't fresh, an arsenic colloid results from the breakdown of the protein, and one thus understands why the food intoxication that occurs is exactly like arsenic poisoning. This was why 'Arsenicum album' was not only the simillimum for the pyelonephritis, but also the 'simile' of the initial energetic imbalance that had probably generated the illness.

At this point I will close this long parenthesis. Such exceptional success occurs rarely today and only with certain rare patients – thank you, Mme Deville! – those who have lived an exceptionally healthy life and have avoided doctors and their medication like the plague. Nowadays unfortunately events take place differently for the majority of those who are ill. Approximate results or failure are the rule, and success the exception. Under these conditions how does the traditional homoeopath behave? He will attribute the failure of his treatment to an imperfect definition of the simillimum and will proceed with a new evaluation of all the symptoms compared to the Materia Medica. This is called 'repertorizing' the symptoms. He is helped in this thankless task by repertories, one of the most famous of which is that of Dr James Tyler Kent, a renowned American professor from the beginning of this century. (Today the more 'up-to-date' doctors delegate this arduous work to the computer.)

This review leads to the choice of a new simillimum which the doctor hopes will be 'truer' than the first and will hopefully bring about a better balance of energies. There will be a real effect if the medication is properly chosen but, as with the first remedy, it won't last very long. And thus the sad game continues: moving from one trial to the next, from remedy to remedy, until doctor and patient are forced to recognize that homoeopathy has become completely ineffective. Some doctors recognize these sad facts sooner than others and go back to using allopathy. Others, more tenacious or headstrong, continue to drag their patients through successive jungles of clinical descriptions, making them purchase quantities of tubes and doses, pills of all sizes to consume month after month and year after year ... These gentlemen's prescriptions are impressive: I've seen some as long as two pages! And the most surprising thing is that the people who sign these amazing shopping lists all say they are partisans of the 'single remedy' approach. (Alas! Even in the early days the master himself railed against his stupid and messy students who were seemingly incapable of finding the correct simillimum!)

There is no point in denying all these failures. But why does such a situation occur? Simply because these stubborn colleagues are unaware of or refuse to accept the concept of energetic blockage so clearly defined by Dr Voll. It is through a close look at the work of his followers that one can discern the way in which homoeopathy will at last be able to emerge from its long period of obscurity. Let us take Senn's school as a model and analyse the technique of one of his students.

A patient comes into the doctor's surgery and sits down in front of his desk. After the usual questioning and discussion of the ineffective (allo- or homoeopathic) treatments attempted to date, the doctor will test the electrical flow of the Chinese meridians. To do this he has the patient hold a tubular electrode in one hand, giving his other hand to the doctor. The doctor then successively places the tip of the other electrode on each of the meridian points on the hand so as to establish contact and close the electrical circuit. Any variance will be considered as a sign of illness. A normal electrical outlet or battery is used and the current isn't usually greater than 0.5mA. Obviously such a weak current isn't felt by the patient, particularly since the existence of the body between the two poles offers resistance, like a tree or a sack of potatoes.

What is amazing, in fact, is that such a ridiculously weak current can pass through this large mass that is so well insulated by the skin. Where then is the 'weak link'? It is precisely in each of those enigmatic acupuncture points that 'pierce' our skin in seven to eight hundred privileged spots linked by the highly individualized lines of force which are called meridians. When the electrode used for testing is applied to one of these points, the electrical current that was interrupted by the resistance of the body is immediately re-established. This can be seen by the sudden jump of the ohmmeter's needle.

Now what exactly does all this mean? The disbelieving colleagues to whom I have often provided demonstrations have volunteered many erroneous explanations. Some imagine that the skin is just thinner at these points; others insist that the skin is never completely dry and that surface perspiration facilitates the passage of electrical current. Others claim that the flow of electrons can occur only if the underlying circulatory system is well irrigated. In fact all these 'explanations' merely seek to deny the immateriality of the meridians. As you will see, these explanations don't stand up very well to an intelligent examination of the phenomenon.

Let us assume that the electrical current is carried by the body fluids once the barrier of the skin has been passed. How then does one explain that on the little finger, for example, the current passes at the originating point of the meridian that corresponds to the small intestine and doesn't at the terminal point of the meridian corresponding to the heart which is less than half an inch away? I have often noticed this with cardiac patients, and I have seen the opposite in the case of typhoid fever, which is very trying for the small intestine. The fact is that no rational explanation of this phenomenon exists if one continues obstinately to deny the existence of the meridians.

Senn and his students systematically study the electrical flow of the meridians. Naturally it is not possible to test all the Chinese acupuncture points, nor even all the meridians. Instead, a standard examination exists that is extremely revealing of the overall state of health of the patient. It involves testing the five fingers of the left or right hand (chosen depending on whether the patient is right- or left-handed). I have already mentioned the two meridians of the little finger, the Heart and Small Intestine. The thumb carries the Lung meridian and the index that of the Large Intestine. These four points already provide information on four organs, and it would be possible to test elsewhere for the others: Liver, Gall Bladder, Kidneys, Bladder, Stomach, Spleen and Pancreas. But the most interesting use of this technique is in the examination of the ring and middle fingers.

The ring finger carries the originating point of a meridian which the Chinese call the 'Triple Heater' (or 'Triple Burner' or 'Triple Energizer') and the middle finger the terminal point of the famous 'Heart Governor' (also called the 'Heart Protector' or the 'Pericardium'), which is the most important of all meridians.

Essentially, these two lines constitute the high-voltage network that supplies current to all the other sectors. Any breakdown in these circuits and illness unquestionably occurs. It may lie hidden, quietly growing, not yet diagnosed or even clearly felt, but the energetic imbalance will already be measurable by the ohmmeter.

This is the materialization of the central phenomenon of any morbid state, the image of the 'disharmony' of vital energy. The visualization of the phenomenon is irrefutable; the electrode is properly applied at the end of the 'Heart Governor' or the beginning of the 'Triple Heater', and yet the current doesn't pass. Here we have the infamous 'blockage' that is the cause of so many failed treatments. Despite years of conscientiously pursued yet none the less futile attempts, the patient can once again take heart and at least hope that the cause of his blockage will be found.

And here we arrive at the moment of truth. With all due respect for Senn, who curiously minimizes in his writings the technique which he himself has helped to disseminate, this search for the cause of the blockage is the key moment of a homoeopathic consultation. As you may well imagine, a thorough questioning is often enough to find the cause of the energetic imbroglio creating the barrier. Most often it turns out to be a vaccination (recent or old), a poorly assimilated childhood illness or some other severe sickness. But, as we saw in the last chapter, the strangest fact of all is that the illness itself, as represented by its nosode, can also be revealed by the ohmmetric test. Dr Senn was able to demonstrate as much at each of his courses.

Let's take a common and simple example: a barrier created by the terrible antitetanus vaccination which has been used and abused by doctors for the last 40 years. The ohmmetric test with the patient is unequivocal: the electric current isn't passing at the 'Heart Governor'. The doctor then has his patient hold a small vial containing the nosode 'Tetanotoxinum' next to the tubular electrode in his left hand. As the other electrode is placed on the 'Heart Governor' point of the right hand, the unbelievable occurs: contact is re-established and the ohmmetric needle regains its normal position. It is as if the energy emitted by the tetanus nosode were able to compensate perfectly the energy deficit created along the 'Heart Governor' by the tetanus vaccine intoxication.

The treatment is logical and childlike in its simplicity: one adequately 'dynamic' oral dose of Tetanotoxinum, and the problem is solved. The effect can be truly radical. With the energetic balance re-established, the patient recovers his health no matter what cause motivated his original illness.

This is how Dr Senn cured innumerable cases in Lausanne designated as incurable and untreatable homoeopathically. You can imagine the miraculous aura in which such spectacular success bathes a doctor! And thus even the most mediocre practitioners of the method managed to glean a few prestigious recoveries.

Unfortunately, these easy triumphs can't deny the other side of the story. Although having thousands of successes to their credit, Voll practitioners have many failures too. This is because the method, elegant as it may be, carries an element of uncertainty, which I will try to explain in the next chapter. This factor is even capable of generating a contrary effect, increasing the energetic disorder and prolonging it indefinitely.

SIX

Technical limits

You have just seen the amazing simplicity with which the ohmmetric technique is able to identify a healing nosode. The example I used was tetanus, one of the most common causes of barriers. The same holds true for diphtheria, polio and vaccinations in general. Infectious illnesses can also create various disturbances that are measurable using Voll's technique. It is nevertheless obvious that, in most cases, the discovery of the electrical disturbance and its related cause is merely a confirmation of the doctor's initial suspicion based on flair, clinical acumen and common sense. Unfortunately there are cases where the cause of illness is far from obvious, being either unknown to the patient himself or rarely encountered by the doctor.

Naturally a very strong temptation exists to let Voll's machine take over the diagnostic process completely. Theoretically you would only need about 50 small bottles to cover most of the morbid possibilities. Passed successively through the patient's hand, the one containing the guilty nosode should sooner or later come to light. All of Voll's students, and Senn the first, have fallen into this trap.

Alas (for those who had thus hoped to be able to avoid the slow process of developing their own sensitivity), the technique is not fully viable in all circumstances. I became aware of this the day that Dr Senn gave me my first demonstration. To explain the method, he began by establishing my energetic profile, and in so doing immediately discovered a blockage at the main meridian. This didn't really surprise me since I had never been very healthy. The details I provided rapidly established an extraordinary history of extremely toxic vaccinations, an unavoidable destiny since I was born in Saigon in the days of French Indochina and spent my childhood in Cambodia. At the time the Institut Pasteur in Saigon ruled tyrannically over the foreign population, 'protecting' it with great care from all possible diseases. We were summoned periodically and submitted to the full range of the Institute's production. This avalanche of exotic toxins was withstood as well as could be expected by my parents and brothers, robust 'carbonics' (homoeopathically the most solid constitutional type). My more fragile 'sodic' heredity unfortunately fared less well. Ten years later, at the end of the war, I apparently still looked like some poor young bird fallen from a nest. In fact, I had never really recovered.

In any event, Dr Senn promptly found cholera, typhus, various typhoid fevers and even yellow fever. With the ohmmeter, each of these tropical nosodes was immediately able to correct the perturbed electrical current. The minute I was home I pulled out all my medical papers to verify the chronology of these first vaccinations. Everything was effectively there, with one exception: yellow fever. My mother confirmed that, since the illness was unknown in Indochina at the time, its prevention wasn't practised and that it had been required only for travellers crossing India following the departure of the British. My only crossing of India had been years before, and then it was with my nose pressed up against the windows of a superb Air France three-engined Dewoitine that after 8 days of flying by sight and a forced landing in the Oman desert had finally brought us safely back to Europe a few weeks before the start of World War II. Since then, I have never been back in the Far East and I have never had a yellow fever vaccination.

Senn's ohmmeter was wrong! This should have been enough warning, but I didn't have the time to think through the possible implications, nor did I have the intelligence to refuse the first proposed treatment. Instead I simultaneously took all the doses that he had given me (since it appeared that all the vaccinations had been contemporaneous, Senn felt this treatment to be appropriate). What a mistake this proved to be! I spent the first night trying as best I could to eliminate the violently re-awakened toxins that my own immunological system had so patiently been working to neutralize over the years. My mentor couldn't have chosen a better way to punish my present disrespect than by unleashing this frightening energetic bombardment on my poor body. Painful as it was, this kind of liberating shock can always be survived. Harder to overcome is the energetic imbroglio that it creates, and that requires infinite therapeutic patience and ingenuity to untangle afterwards. I never saw Dr Senn again as a patient, and although it took me 4 years of laborious groping to restore my lost equilibrium, it was from this lesson that I formed the basis of my own therapeutic method.

Later you will hear more about the subtle mechanisms of this error that I have since baptized the 'Mikado effect'. But for the moment I will return to the first mistake: the ohmmeter's condemnation of an innocent nosode. I went back through each step of the process used. First Senn had tested 'Cholera'. The needle on the machine had immediately jumped, my main meridian was freed and the barrier was broken. The same liberating power was then attributed to all the nosodes he subsequently tested, even though the barrier momentarily displaced by the 'Cholera' nosode was not yet back in place. If the experiment had been started with the yellow fever nosode instead, the needle would not have moved.

It seemed to me that this was clearly a case of the mysterious and still controversial phenomenon called remanence that troubles so many radiesthesists. For my part I have seen its indirect effects too frequently to deny its existence. In fact, I honestly must confess to a passion for this medically unorthodox area, which I have been studying and experimenting with for the last 20 years. I have never tired of the lessons in humility that it brings to our academic vanity.

I told my teacher of this reasoning, but he was unwilling to accept it. So I continued alone with my experimental critique of Voll's method and soon discovered an anomaly of some interest. Naturally I had acquired an ohmmeter at the outset of my homoeopathic apprenticeship. Senn had each of his students buy a small transistorized version developed by a young university researcher. One of my first concerns was to test the meridians of my patients to get a feeling for their energetic balance, and thus their real state of health and potential receptivity to a homoeopathic treatment.

It quickly became apparent that all my chronically ill patients had classic barriers on the main meridians. During the rest of 1975 I energetically tracked down the nosodes that would unblock them, and was not surprised to find that they were most frequently those of common vaccinations and childhood illnesses. However, unlike Senn and his other students, I was constantly finding that once a liberating nosode had unblocked a barrier, I could put as many other nosodes as I wished into the hands of my patients, but the initial barrier would not reappear. It didn't matter whether the experiment lasted a minute or half an hour, the effect was always the same. In addition, after the tests it seemed that the patient's vital energy had been rebalanced in a durable way. It was as if the simple act of placing the correct element in the patient's hand had instantaneously provided the missing quantum of energy. In fact, I was being told more and more frequently that the current could actually be felt, either as a warm sensation in the hand holding the electrode or as a tingling or even a shock in certain fingertips. Even more interesting was the fact that, once a successful detection had occurred, it became completely impossible for me to use this easy technical method to find other eventual barriers or their cause. No matter whether a day, 6 weeks or 6 months passed: the surprising results of the first day almost always remained. The patient's vital energy seemed to have been reactivated once and for all! In short, it was only rarely that I discovered new Vollian blockages in a patient tested successfully the first time.

This observation confirmed the idea of remanence, but it also introduced a new element: the unusual duration of this enigmatic phenomenon. At first I thought it might be the machine. During Dr Senn's vacation I inherited his original Vollian equipment and proceeded to redo all my tests. In vain! There were no more barriers than when I used my own little battery-driven machine. But Senn and the other students were able to detect new barriers daily using this same equipment.

Since it wasn't the tool that was creating the remanence, and it logically couldn't be the patients themselves since they were obviously all different from each other, there was only one remaining characteristic common to all the tests: me! I had to admit that each time I was measuring, I was unable to prevent my own energy from interfering with the electrical phenomena being measured. In fact, I had been finding myself to be abnormally exhausted each evening and had been unable to find any explanation until I recognized and acknowledged my patients' involuntary 'vampirism'. At the time I didn't understand how this was taking place, but everything seemed to indicate that my patients' energy deficits, once diminished by the correct nosode, were being lastingly compensated by a current emanating directly from myself, modulated by the machine and taking effect before the oral absorption of the appropriate remedy. One would have said that, by the simple fact of my placing into the patient's hand the witness to be tested, I had spontaneously catapulted into his deficient energetic circuits a quantum of correcting energy from my hand, modulated by the witness.

But, better still, I had never had to change the batteries of my machine despite daily use over a period of 9 years, whilst my almost unused back-up ohmmeter often failed me because of its run-down batteries. I have to admit an even more startling fact: when my ohmmeter's batteries began to give signs of weakness, noticed during the daily testings, this unfailingly announced a drop in my own vitality, a passing weakness or the flu. At these moments I find barriers in everyone. Then when I have recovered my normal health, my patients' barriers magically disappear, and simultaneously the battery in the apparatus is miraculously recharged! It seems that my energy apparently indulges itself in the activation of the energy systems of inert objects as well as human beings. Could it be that in biology, like in experimental physics, the observer modifies the observed phenomenon solely by his own presence?

A fourth, and now almost daily, observation tends to support this supposition. The patients tested by Dr Senn or his students, and pronounced severely deficient energetically, somehow acquired a satisfactory balance with me even before I had started seeking the appropriate nosode. Of course I found small indications of energetic blockage, but they were so small that the ohmmeter's needle barely moved. It was as if my physical presence alone was enough to alter the results of the tests. My personal energy was somehow helping to erase the energetic deficits of these patients.

During these first experiments I discovered another troubling electrical property of the Chinese meridians. It suffices to introduce any healthy person into the ohmmetric circuit of the patient and all trace of electrical imbalance disappears! I illustrated this discovery to Dr Senn by involving him directly in a demonstration. At the time (1976), he presented a serious blockage of the 'Heart Governor', which by his own confession had resisted all efforts of elimination. I took his left hand in my right hand, took the mass electrode myself in my left hand, and with the same hand tested his right hand with the exploring electrode held by its isolating casing. The blockage vanished instantaneously! I had managed to establish what electricians call a serial connection.

It is also possible to multiply the number of people in the chain. I've tried it with my whole family, and the current passes through everyone, like the multicoloured garlands you see at fun fairs. The experiment would be worth trying on a really big scale to find out if there is a maximum number that the circuit can accommodate. I do know that certain esoteric groups use hand-holding techniques for collective vitalization that are based on the same principle, and which are said to be therapeutically effective on an individual level.

But this series of discoveries was shortly to put me into an embarrassing situation. Senn's fundamental lessons had made me into a perfect Vollian disciple. Like the other pupils and the master himself, I should have spent the rest of my life seeking barriers, and by using the machine, easily identifying the correct nosode to remove them. Unfortunately, my curious physiological disposition was apparently going to prohibit any instrumentation help to me. I later came to understand this phenomenon as being a function of what can be called my 'aura', which was pulling the weakened astral bodies of my patients along in the wake of its own energy. Needless to say, this kind of 'higher' reality is a little hard for a Western doctor to accept easily.

Since I was unwilling to let myself become entangled in esoteric complexities, I set out to find some kind of practical solution to this mechanical impasse. And in 1976 I found it through a reference by my teacher to Dr Constantine Hering. This German doctor, born on the first day of the 19th century, had been told by his thesis director to study Hahnemann in order subsequently to combat his theories. Now, as always happens to awakened intelligence, the truth of the homoeopathic principles imposed itself on his critical analysis with such force that he very soon became the most ardent defender of this method! Hering was, without doubt, the most brilliant disciple of the master (who he never met personally), and he was to make an invaluable contribution to the international dissemination of homoeopathic methods through his exemplary successes. Following his emigration to the United States, he trained many adepts and created the first American Homoeopathic Academy.

Hahnemann owes his immortality to the codification of the Law of Similarity. But Hering's definition of the law that now bears his name is no less of a contribution. It can be stated as follows:

> Illness evolves from the periphery towards the centre, from exterior to interior. The process of recovery is exactly the opposite and moves from centre to periphery, from inside to outside.

The scope of this dictum is universal. Hering's Law is as applicable to allopathy as it is to homoeopathy and yet it remains unknown to medical teachers and thus to their students. It nevertheless irresistibly determines the destiny of all illnesses, and without its acceptance no doctor can be in a position to promise lasting recovery to his patients.

Like all brilliant ideas, through its simplicity it is accessible to good old common sense. And in fact, as I have explained these principles to my patients over the years, I have found that the common sense of the man in the street accepts without the slightest difficulty the notion that a bad case of measles is only fully cured if it has really 'come out', while more academic intelligences tend to be far more reticent towards the idea. But the supreme audacity of this law is that it claims to govern not only the 'topographical' expression of the illness, but the chronological evolution as well. For example, an abscess spontaneously heals by bursting at the skin surface. This local progression is visible and not very mysterious. What also needs to be known is that an infant's milk rash evolves into a child's eczema and often then into an adult's asthma. The worsening is chronological as well as topographical. Over the years the illness has worsened by leaving the skin – the surface – and moving into the body. Hering's law directs that the resultant internal illness, asthma, can be fully cured only by leaving the body through the skin, momentarily recreating the eczematous condition of the child and the scabby condition of the baby. Recovery can be accomplished only by strictly respecting the reversed spatiotemporal order.

It is this chronological aspect of Hering's Law that interested me as I tried to find a solution to the impasse created by my inability to use Voll's machine. As you will see, a very simple thought process finally solved the problem.

Let us take the case of one of my patients who had an unfortunate tendency to come down frequently with various colds or often with bronchitis. I see cases like this almost daily. From our perspective, this obvious drop in general resistance to infection comes from a permanent imbalance in the patient's vital energy, which had been 'put out of tune' (this is the term used by Hahnemann himself) by one or several past events. For our example, let us imagine that at the age of 10 the patient had a bad reaction to a BCG (tuberculosis) vaccination followed by a bad case of scarlet fever at the age of 15. In our terms, we would say that the shock of the vaccination had created an important imbalance of the vital energy at 10 years, and the scarlet fever a second shock and further imbalance at the age of 15. Suppose, at 20 years, the patient is examined by a student of Voll's method. The doctor will not have any difficulty with the ohmmeter in finding the electrical trace of these two events on the 'Heart Governor', which, like the Lung meridian, will in all probability be blocked. The treatment will naturally have to respect the chronological order of these illnesses in order to re-establish the harmony that was disturbed when they occurred. This is simple enough to understand. The doctor will first give the Scarlatina nosode, which will repair the shock at 15 years , then the BCG nosode, which will erase the one at 10 years. This harmless isopathic treatment can, in this precise case, give to our young man a perfect energetic balance, and the distressing morbid tendency will disappear as by enchantment! This example respects Hering's Law perfectly.

But let us suppose for a moment that the same patient, while recovering from scarlet fever at 15 years, had fallen and suffered from a slight concussion, so slight that it was forgotten and never even mentioned to the doctor. In addition, let us imagine that at 16 years the same person had remained in bed for about a week with 'some kind of flu' with signs of meningitis. This, too, was judged too insignificant to be mentioned. The doctor is thus completely unaware of these two events, both of which had the potential to create further energetic imbalance. The prescribed treatment naturally remains the same as outlined above, but the violence of the patient's reaction and the inefficiency of the treatment leave the doctor perplexed and disturbed. What has happened?

The answer is clear, as I am sure you have already guessed; the treatment quite simply didn't respect Hering's Law. He should have started with the incident of 16 years, the so-called 'flu', then the concussion, then the scarlet fever, then the BCG, and then the treatment would have succeeded. The failure to respect the chronology had liberated energies that were in fact subservient to other energies that themselves remained blocked. Thus the subtle skein of the temporal continuity of vital energy had inadvertently been entangled. I have familiarly baptized this hitch of the Voll method the 'Mikado effect' that I mentioned earlier.

Perhaps you remember the childhood game where a handful of sticks of different values is thrown haphazardly in a heap on the table. The objective is to remove them one by one from the pile without moving any others. Children who are impatient, greedy, near-sighted or clumsy all regularly fall into the trap of pulling at the most visible, highest valued or what they perceive to be the easiest stick to pull out. And the whole carefully balanced edifice comes tumbling down.

This is exactly what happened to me that autumn day in 1975 when my treatment started in my new teacher's surgery. In his haste to find the key element, Dr Senn didn't take the time to establish clearly the chronology of my medical history and paid attention only to the most intensely energetic events such as cholera, typhus and yellow fever. Voll's machine had certainly been 'short-sighted', with the resultant clumsy treatment that had liberated such an extraordinary array of reactions from the depths of my childhood, ignoring the many other destabilizing events of 40 years of my life. In a word, he had blatantly violated Hering's Law, the key law to the art of healing.

I paid for this mistake very dearly, since, as I mentioned earlier, it took me 4 years and the patience of Job to unravel the energetic imbroglio thus created, just like a poor knitter who loses precious time trying to untangle, one by one, the tangle of knots in her wool, caused by the antics of a playful kitten.

In my misfortune, I received help from an unexpected direction in the form of medical files that accompanied the patients sent to me by my teacher. It was easy to draw a parallel between their situation and mine. Indeed, the patients who most systematically presented anomalies in my ohmmetric tests were those he sent me with the fallacious guarantee that they wouldn't burden my already heavy schedule for long, since he had constantly followed their cases for the last 10 or 20 years, some even since their childhood!

It is through the minute study of their case histories that I understood the reason for their strangely incurable nature despite the attentive care of such a reputed doctor. The reason being, of course, the repeated violations of Hering's Law. These repeated infractions the doctor had naturally perpetrated without malice, but by simple ignorance of important events in their history – events that did not have enough impact on the energetic balance to leave traces that were measurable on the ohmmeter.

It is really this lack of sensitivity of detection that is at the heart of the problem with energetic medicine. Voll's students speak of blocks and barriers and believe they can 'see' them with their machines. But the present technology is not yet totally reliable. Certain electrical configurations are deemed blockage by some and normal by others and some signs are considered normal by all which in all likelihood are misleading.

The only way to get to the truth is through unprejudiced, rational thinking. But it is a waste of time to continue talking about 'distortions', 'deviations', 'barriers'. The one and only object of the study of medicine that heals is the radiant splendour of vital energy, assuring health through its harmonious balance. We must in the final reckoning have the audacity to ask the one question of real interest, the only truly intelligent question:

'Vital energy, who are you?'

SEVEN

Vital energy

Readers in a hurry, or knowledgeable in the field, might feel that reading the present chapter would be a waste of time. In fact if they so wish they can proceed immediately to Chapter 9, the real heart of this work. They will find there the detailed outline of the therapy, the practical end result of a reasoning process as simple as it is pretentious.

Simple it most certainly is. Even a high school student can grasp it. And pretentious too, as a man must have a fairly healthy dose of naive ambition to attempt a definition of life itself. But to speak of 'vital energy' is nothing less than to use superfluous words to describe this primary aspect of life, which is, simply, 'energy'. We will see that the real problem with medicine is semantics, a problem of definitions, a more or less amusing war of words in which the only arbitrator will be your own common sense.

Let us start at the beginning – the definition of medicine. The answer is simple and clear: it is the art of re-establishing and conserving health. Since health is nothing more than a quality of life, in its turn we have first to define 'life'.

Open your dictionaries. They all agree on the essential idea: 'life is an energy that animates inert matter'. Let us call this energy 'vital energy'. Hahnemann called it '*dynamis*'; others called it 'ethereal fluid', 'vital principle', etc. Whatever it may be called, the essential character remains the same: vital energy is a force that animates inert matter.

This is the same as saying that matter, under the effect of this force, loses its inertia. It moves. Moving means changing places, and a change in place is a movement that brings an object from one place to another. Thus movement inherently implies the fundamental notion of space. But the move from one place to another isn't instantaneous, there is a time-lapse from the departure to the arrival. And thus we reach another fundamental notion: time. So moving means changing places in space and in time. This is what can be seen in the spectacle of inert matter animated by vital energy. It propagates in space – it grows; it matures and endures over time – it ages. It even manages to reproduce itself once certain thresholds of spatial growth and temporal maturity have been reached.

So vital energy is: 'a force that moves matter in space and time'. This is how one can describe its animating power. But now let us take a closer look at the object of this action: matter. What in fact is this seemingly common thing called matter? Here we have the question that over the centuries has been the major business of our sciences as they have tried to help us understand life through our senses. Ever since the discovery of the molecular structure of matter, our knowledge has taken giant steps forward. Everyone today knows that molecules consist of atoms, and all secondary school students know the periodic table of the elements, that fabulous register of all atoms.

This leads on to the next obvious question: what is an atom? Now here the answer is considerably less clear. Everyone knows that an atom is made up of a central core and of surrounding electrons, but the nature of these electrons as well as the elements of the central core remains mysterious for most of us. Don't worry, I am not planning to subject you to a course in physics! I must however remind you that, ever since Max Planck and the appearance of quantum physics, the ultimate constituent parts of matter appear progressively with each new theory to be less and less 'material'. Indeed, thanks to our scientists, we now know that matter itself is also energy.

Now this is quite an amusing turn of events, since, if you remember, my first definition of vital energy was energy animating matter. Well, since matter itself is energy, vital energy must therefore be an energetic system animating another energetic system. And since animating means moving something in space and time, our definition now has to become: 'vital energy is an energetic system that moves another energetic system in space and time'.

Obviously any system capable of moving another one imposes itself by what we must assume to be a greater force. In effect one might say that one system is therefore superior and somehow directs the other. In any event, what should be retained is the fact that the space and time in which this movement occurs can be directly observed and measured. In fact they represent the restricted area within which science operates in its attempts to explain the universe. And what is prodigiously interesting, what gives charm to our age, is that, at every attempt to escape this framework, philosophical and mathematical thought inevitably leads us back to the same troubling and essential bipolarity of space and time. Today everyone knows that, following the demonstration that matter is energy, quantum physics now shows us that energy itself is merely the cloak of light worn by time as it moves through space. In the jargon of mathematics, energy loses its name and becomes the 'space-time continuum' – an enigmatic entity whose primary characteristic, indissociability, would be far too cumbersome to try to explain here. What we must remember is that time becomes the fourth dimension of space. This semantic sleight of hand is called a 'spatiotemporal equation' and can be verified by calculation. This is prodigious and brings us back once again to our definition of vital energy. Logically, it now becomes: 'vital energy is a superior energetic system that moves an inferior energetic system (the space–time continuum) in visible space and measurable time'.

Do you follow me? You have to admit that the reasoning is not very difficult. But it is going to become so soon, as the next, unavoidable, question will bring us to the crux of the problem: 'What then is the nature of this superior system which can impose itself with such mastery over the space–time continuum?' Now this is indeed a sticky problem. I have to admit that I have never seen this question asked in a medical treatise, and our scholars themselves, heirs to rational and materialist scientific thought, have been too busy over the last half-century exploring only the space–time continuum itself, the true face of matter. Doctors, more practical than scientific, are still exploring the directly measurable space and time in front of their noses. You can therefore easily imagine that with the entire scientific community thus stuck in the exploration of inferior realities, no one is interested in taking on the burden of any superior realities! Doctors therefore never pose themselves this fundamental question. However, the superior energetic system clearly exists since we are all alive, and pathfinder scholars will soon help us, indirectly, to understand better its nature.

But first, let us think. What could this superior force be that commands space and time? Can a power exist that can bring to heel two such noble and lofty concepts? Just thinking about them alone makes the mind reel, with one leading to infinity and the other to eternity. And they let themselves be dominated? Is there a word in our scientific vocabulary to designate such a power? I don't think one exists, since we all know that no one has the power to limit space or stop time.

At this point the answer becomes obvious: any power dominating the space–time continuum must also be related to infinity and eternity, must belong to the same family. It can only be another space–time continuum! Isn't it logical that this superior energy should itself be space and time like its inferior namesake, matter? The calculations of quantum physics apply to the concept of energy itself without reference to any superior or inferior position.

But the latter is precisely my present concern, since my first definition is now so simplified as to appear redundant: 'vital energy is a superior space–time continuum that moves an inferior space-time continuum'. As you can see, the nature of these two terms is rigorously identical. The only way out of this vicious circle is the qualitative difference. Of the two protagonists, one is superior, the other inferior. They are of the same family, but the first dominates the second. The superior must therefore possess an additional authority or strength. And here we are back at the beginning, unable to clarify further the ultimate question: where does this extra power come from? This is where I reach the limits of my intellectual ability, and, not being a scholar, must seek the desired answers through the intelligence of humility – simple common sense.

The first solution that comes to mind could be imagined as follows. The extra power of the superior continuum comes from an additional quality that the inferior continuum doesn't possess. It could perhaps be a fifth dimension which one day might be explained through calculations. But not everyone has the means to reason outside the usual channels of thought, and certain mathematicians, even in the West, can end up in mental asylums.

A second, and more modest, solution appeals to me more than the first. The superior continuum does have a particular although not exclusive quality which it shares with the inferior continuum. This quality is therefore necessarily variable. And what kind of variability is possible for a four-dimensional continuum? The first three dimensions seem to be identical in both systems since it is hard to imagine how infinity could be greater in one than in the other. The variable quality can therefore affect only the fourth dimension, that of time. Intuitively we all have a confirmation of this idea through our experience of differing perceptions of time passing depending on the associated emotional content of waiting: intense joy or deadly boredom.

Curiously, physics was not very interested in the concept of time until the beginning of quantum physics. But, ever since the work of Ilya Prigogine, scholars have been paying time more attention. Very roughly summarized, their speculations point towards a probability that there are several speeds of time. It would therefore seem reasonable in my definition of vital energy to attribute a greater speed to the time of the superior continuum.

In the material world the greatest possible speed is given by Einstein's famous equation – $E=mc^2$. This gives c as the speed of light in the void, which is assumed to be a constant. For as long as physicians believed in a limit to speed, it was impossible to imagine anything beyond this frontier. But the students of Nicola Tesla have shown that the void is perhaps not as empty as everyone thought, and the famous constant is something less than invariable. The naive amongst us can follow this easily since we know that thought moves faster than any photons. This is why we can accept without mental contortions the idea that, in the animated universe, the superior continuum can impose itself on the temporal world of these photons. Not only is it faster, it is instantaneous, it is thought itself.

You see, I have just made a leap myself. This pirouette, the classical inversion of the hunted hunter, has been dictated by my right brain because the left brain has lost control of the game. This is a miniature version of the conflict occurring in today's science, and is called a paradigm shift – an enormous upheaval that forces us to abandon our old systems of reference and antiquated dogmas, replacing them with more functional intellectual schemas. This new guiding model has been prefigured by all of us in our right brains, the source of all analogical and synthetic thought. Its message is imperious – and so simple! It tells us that the enigmatic concept of space and time exists solely through our awareness of its existence. Indeed, how can one refuse to admit that time and space exist only for those who measure them?

Perhaps you think this is nonsense since, after all, the universe existed before man's appearance on Earth. But the consciousness that I am talking about is not our exclusive privilege. The most intelligent men on our planet have accepted the idea that long before the appearance of any form of life, there was an existence of space and time through the 'consciousness' of the first constituent elements of matter! In the famous equation $E=mc^2$, space–time is defined in relation to the photon, that enigmatic central character that is apparently aware of its destiny and retains the memory of its distant past. Once again advanced physics surprises us with its extremely serious assurance that electrons themselves are capable of action, thought, knowledge ... and even love!

One could hardly call this the dry language of mathematics. In this leap beyond itself, physics has become metaphysics. At last scholars realize that the only way to knowledge is through this great leap, thus confirming André Malraux's prediction that the 21st century 'would either be mystical or there won't be a 21st century'.

Through the introduction of consciousness into its equations, science has at last linked itself to the ancient truth of the Tao, as Fritjof Capra so aptly describes. In so doing, it has authorized the most extreme audacity in my laborious concern for a definition. What does our vital energy become in this new paradigm? We have seen that it is space–time, and also superior to matter since faster than light. If there is a consciousness of matter, this one must be far superior since it represents the awakening of matter itself!

Who are you, vital energy? My final answer, in the form of a Zen koan, is as follows: you are infinite space, maintained in a subjective point by the instantaneous nature of time as experienced by the consciousness of the subject. That point is you, me, all of us. It is the animal, our brother, the plant, our sister and even the stone or the electron, all individual entities, but also completely interdependent, bound together in an indissoluble cosmic unity, governed by Him, Him Who Is.

EIGHT

The central problem: transmission

All the great civilizations preceding ours have produced great doctors. History gives us some rare accounts of their achievements and also shows us that theology was never far from their preoccupations. In fact, most of the time the leading doctor of any given dynasty in power was also high priest of the dominant religion. This situation lasted for centuries.

In the West the dominating explosion of Greek rationalism, an incomplete shadow of the fabulous science of Egypt, gradually took away from theology its royal power over all areas of knowledge and finally led to the triumph of rational materialism, which rules our universities today.

Our civilization is totally materialistic. God is no longer the driving force behind laws or government and is no longer taught to architects, chemists or engineers, let alone to teachers or economists. Among the most serious of errors, God is completely absent from medical amphitheatres. He is the One by whose universal consciousness space and time escape from the void. Vital energy, to whom we owe life, is only one of the more flamboyant aspects of His total consciousness through which the universe exists. Although in the preceding chapter I was unable to contribute much to advance the study of His incommensurable greatness, I was obliged at least to point to the origin of life as a prelude to speaking of health. What you will read here, perhaps with surprise, will not be found in other medical treatises. But it is essential that you recognize that no further therapeutic progress will take place without constant reference to the laws by which vital energy transmits life to matter.

Laws? I should probably write the Law, since there is only one law which presides over the manifestations of primal energy.

Edgar Cayce, the greatest of all clairvoyants, called it several times the Law of the One. I was receptive to his message, and propose to demonstrate here that life cannot be explained in more than one way. If you have followed me thus far, you have recognized that vital energy is in essence divine. But this understanding has not necessarily enabled you to visualize it clearly. In order to do this, you must make it perceptible to your senses, give it a form.

The form of an energy, no matter what its nature, is always described in modern physics as a wave. Whether we are examining a stone thrown into water or the trajectory of atomic particles, the movement created always takes the form of a wave. This is perfectly logical, for don't forget that all energy is space and time. To show this continuum on paper, classical physics always depicts the passage of time with an abscissa (the horizontal or *x*-coordinate) and expanding space with an ordinate (the vertical or *y*-coordinate). Graphically, the resulting sinusoid (sine wave curve) immediately reveals the nature of the energy represented as characterized by the wavelength, amplitude and frequency. In this manner, a form can be given to the full range of known physical energies whether they animate galaxies or atoms. But we will not find vital energy in this material range. As we have seen, it does not align itself with the inferior space–time continuum. It controls it! It is itself superior space–time, lifted up by the elevation of its own degree of consciousness.

Since a sinusoidal curve was acceptable for depiction of the inferior materiality, nothing opposes its use in the superior context. But, rather than joining this new sinusoid to the first, it will instead be placed on top. The resulting image of two superposed waves immediately brings to mind the astrological symbol for the constellation and age of Aquarius. This is an example of disconcerting foresight on the part of the ancient Sumerian scholars who perhaps knew that our troubled period, on Aquarius's threshold, would finally lead to the rediscovery of energetic harmony.

This double-wave symbol, a wonderful image of vital energy in action, is totally irreplaceable. No other image could be more suggestive or concise about the real nature of the central enigma of our lives. At a glance it is obvious that we are dealing with the transfer of energy, of information. The central problem of life is simply a problem of transmission. The superior wave leaves its

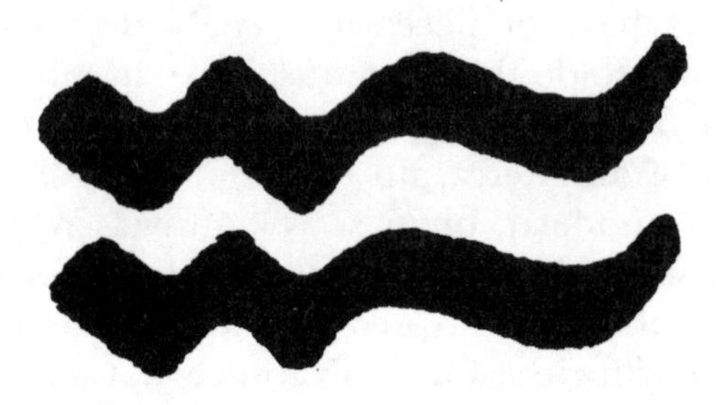

The double-wave symbol

imprint on the inferior one, giving it form and rhythm, modelling it exactly.

How does this transmission take place? You will understand immediately if you have ever seen a musician play a viola d'amore, that instrument with a double set of chords where one set vibrates while a bow is pulled over the other. Or perhaps you have performed the physics experiment with two tuning forks, where one is instantaneously activated by activating the other. In these classic examples, physics easily explains what is taking place. A series of sound waves initiated by the movement spreads into the surrounding environment – the air – which becomes the supporting mechanism for the energy emitted and thus formally transmits it to a sensitive receptor. If you remove the intermediary, – the air for example – the transmission fails.

All energy transmissions respect the same schema: a wave of

movement, a vibrating medium, an induced wave. In the range of waves identified by physics, the vibrating medium is assimilated to a field: an electric field, magnetic field, etc. What does this notion mean? Simply that energy being carried doesn't follow a single straight line like a cord tied between two poles. It spreads out in all directions in space where it can be seen and measured at any moment, and naturally in the two senses of time as well, don't forget!

How can one visualize this vibrating, four-dimensional medium? In endless ways! Imagine what you wish: a very elastic mass, a cushion of air, a shock absorber, a jelly pudding or whatever. The important thing to know is that whatever energy is applied to any side of this mass will automatically be transmitted to the other sides. This transmission can occur through various channels or lines of force, which will be more or less direct and rapid depending on the resistance encountered inside the vibrating medium.

These innumerable channels are like threads woven into a kind of flexible pattern supporting the most wonderful fabric of all: our life. Life is nothing else than the spatio-temporal transmission of superior energy, immaterial and divine, to the very material energy of the lower space–time continuum. And health can now be defined very simply as the perfect harmony of this transmission. If disorder takes the place of this harmony, the pleasure of living disappears and illness sets in.

But if you are tired out by this four-dimensional reasoning let us go back to the symbol of Aquarius since it will help you to understand that there can be three causes of illness and that medicine can in turn act at three different levels. One possible cause for our earthly miseries could be a flaw in the superior wave. In my view this is the origin of the illnesses referred to as karmic, and recognized by oriental medicine, which is more subtle than our own. With these illnesses, only an intervention at the higher energetic level can bring about a cure. Christ was a master of the art, as are the Kahuna priests of Polynesia and competent witchdoctors of certain so-called primitive tribes. But a detailed study of these perfectly comprehensible phenomena goes beyond the scope of this book.

A second and very commonplace cause won't retain our attention much longer than the first; it is the physical alteration of the lower wave – broken legs, perforated ulcers, clogged veins, a proliferation of malignant cells, etc. All these attacks on our corporal integrity are called lesional, and are less a concern of medicine since they are better handled through surgery. What a splendid revenge for surgeons who were for so long held in contempt and treated like barbers by other doctors!

The real area where our doctors' talents can be exercised is therefore in between these two extreme waves. To simplify this image even further, you can imagine the two energetic poles as two interlocking wheels, the superior activating the inferior with the space between the cogs representing the zone in which medicine can operate. The drama of our hi-tech Western medicine is its complete servitude to chemistry; of all the innumerable paths criss-crossing the intermediate zone, our doctors have recognized only the physiopathological ones discovered by biochemists. Continuing the mechanical image used above, it is as if our doctors were mechanics putting oil (naturally of the best quality) between the two interlocking wheels. Through this lubrication they avoid the inevitable small jamming and blockage of the machine and are proud of their 'exploits'. But in so doing they are committing a fatal error, and one that a good mechanic wouldn't make. A meticulous worker, master of his trade, knows that from time to time the oil in the gearbox has to be completely changed. But our doctors, servants to the pharmaceutical industry, don't have this professional conscience, and will continue to add oil for ever without ever purging the motor. And their patients, those with hypertension, heart problems, rheumatism, depression, allergies or cancer, will remain ignorant of the enormous risk they are taking and will put up with lifetimes of pills and injections. Oil polluted by the inevitable waste products will never be purged. And one day a cog in the lower wheel breaks, transmission stops and death is avoided only if the surgeon arrives in time to either fix the gears or change the wheel.

This is not what one would call enlightened medicine, and the public is not taken in. Of course lubrication is sometimes necessary, and I too use certain palliative treatments. But the primary obligation of a doctor is to heal, to re-establish the harmony of the energetic transmission through all its channels.

For this to happen the existence of these multiple channels must first be recognized. A real doctor has to study them without limiting himself to the biochemical exploration taught in medical schools. By restricting medical research to the meanderings of chemistry over the last 50 years, our professors bear the heavy responsibility of retarding the accession to good health by the population at large. Millions of deaths and useless misfortunes could have been avoided if it had been recognized in time that chemistry itself is only a subchapter of particle physics. The drama is that this is still not recognized even today, and the Nobel Prize for medicine continues to be given to people who are really only brilliant chemists!

But luckily times are changing. The enormous hecatomb of cancer victims and cardiovascular illness has aroused both public opinion and the entire scientific community. At last health appears to be too precious to be entrusted solely to the doctors. It has become obvious for an attentive public that medical progress can take place only through the exploration of the entire biophysical network of which biochemistry is just a part.

I discussed some of these ways in the first chapter. In Ménétrier's biological catalysis, as in new dietetic techniques, the transfer of information occurs through ionic exchange. In tissue therapy, it takes place at a molecular level according to a physical code of which doctors have never even heard. And in certain subtle manipulative techniques, the biophysical regulation is even more telling. The fact is that today's most exciting work in medical research is being directed by mathematicians and physicists. The most interesting book on therapy in general that I have read recently was written by a physicist, Dr Charles Terreaux. If you suffer from migraine, anxiety or depression, you will learn how to cure yourself simply by modifying nutritionally the physical parameters of the forces at work in your stomach, in battle with its contents. The most intelligent book I have read recently on molecular biology was written by a mathematician, Dr Etienne Guillé, who does not hesitate to call on radiesthesia to decipher the secrets of DNA. The most interesting ideas about the art of healing are no longer to be found in medical journals, but instead in articles of a general scientific scope that can be purchased at the local bookshop. And the list is growing daily, from Vincent's already old bioelectronics to the more modern Mora-therapy of the German electrotechnicians, or to any of the new 'lay' pioneers of tomorrow's medicine. They all have one thing in common: the primacy of homoeopathy and acupuncture in the regulation of the transmission of energy, the key to health.

As I studied acupuncture for only 3 years I am not in a position to speak about it with authority. It is homoeopathy that I now want to present to you for what it is in reality: the royal road permitting the easy transfer from the higher order to the lower material world.

You will remember Hahnemann's definition of illness. He always used the term 'out of tune'. This literally means 'lack of harmony': the inferior wave does not vibrate in unison with the higher wave. The network of innumerable biophysical paths which link them together in wavelength, amplitude and known or unknown frequencies, is momentarily distorted, deformed. The current no longer passes. If the distortion in the network is minor, the suppleness of the system usually allows contact to be rapidly re-established. This is an example of acute benign illness. If the deformation is brutal and severe, the acute illness can become serious and even fatal. In both cases the inferior wave is not vibrating in a synchronized way. And in both cases a homoeopathic treatment is both simple and efficient. The doctor must identify the precise nature of the distortion as it is revealed through signs and symptoms, and, through the 'portrait gallery', find the most similar remedy that is capable of provoking the same disfunction. If found correctly and quickly, the right remedy will put the inferior wave back into phase.

But illness is not often this simple; the multi-informational network that joins the two undulating poles is rarely a perfect conductor. Its numerous paths are not neatly lined up one beside the other like well-combed fibres in a woven cloth. Instead there are a multitude of distortions and deformations, the traces of the many mishaps of our lives. Since the network is itself space and time, like the two poles it joins, the alterations that it undergoes can be seen in its spatial and temporal traces. This is like saying that events that were important enough to leave marks or distortions are somehow kept in a ledger or memorized by the network itself. The picture of these distortions, revealed by the diagnosis of the moment, is merely the composite result of all the distortions undergone in the past – a bit like a suddenly knotted shoelace created by your own clumsy or impatient movements.

You can now understand why if it is to be efficient, treatment must correct the distortion in both time and space. The knots have to be untangled. But no chemical treatment has the property of being able to act in both time and space simultaneously. This feat is the great speciality of homoeopathic remedies, recognized by so few doctors and underexploited even by many homoeopaths. These remedies have the power to vibrate simultaneously in all four dimensions of space and time. And this can be demonstrated!

The demonstration of this fact is the purpose of Part II of the present work, which will present a collection of cures made possible by this wonderful property in every medical field. But, for those readers who are interested in experimentally verifying these assertions themselves, I will outline below a few steps that can be followed and reproduced at little cost. First, purchase three remedies at the pharmacy; one representing each of the categories of matter: animal, vegetable or mineral. For example, you could choose Apis, Aconitum and Zincum. You will need three tubes containing remedies which have been 'potentized' to a low level (for instance, the fourth centesimal potency, written in shorthand as 4C, or simply 4 (*see* Glossary)), and three other tubes with the same remedies at a more powerful level (12C). A third set of tubes containing neutral pills will be needed as a control in the experiment. The next step is to find an amateur photographer who practises the Kirlian technique. (Developed in 1945 by a Russian couple, this technique consists of photographing subjects that have been placed in a high frequency electrical field.) It should not be too difficult to find people familiar with the method as it has been widely disseminated and commercialized in many cities.

The next step is easy. Place one potentized and one neutral pill on photographic paper and take their picture. Do this for each remedy in both of its potencies. The result is remarkable! While the control pill remains consistently identical in all cases, the others are all significantly different from each other and surrounded by a surprisingly large halo. Further, the corona of light varies depending on the animal, vegetable or mineral origin of the remedy. In my opinion a serious study of this phenomenon would enable the up-to-now impossible identification of homoeopathic remedies. In fact, I don't understand why the major firms don't publish a photographic atlas of key remedies as an aid to the study of their biophysical properties.

But one of the most important aspects of the Kirlian experiment is the very marked difference that exists between the low and high potencies of each remedy. The halo around a 12C is clearly much bigger than that of a 4C. In itself this should at the very least be sufficient proof to put an end to the hostility levelled at homoeopathy for almost 2 centuries by orthodox medical practitioners. Yet today one can still hear them on television and read their declarations in the press stating that homoeopathy works owing to a placebo effect and that potentization is merely the verbiage of charlatans. Such stubborn academic dogmatism makes them perfect partners for the learned men who demonstrated to Galileo that the earth could not possibly be round.

These experiments are easily reproduced and confirm some of the highly sophisticated bases of Raman-laser spectrophotometry and anthroposophic research into crystallization. All these avant-garde studies tend to prove one thing with certainty: the homoeopathic remedy does expand into different spatial directions and does leave a trace. It is thus able to distort one of the fundamental biophysical structures of vital energy and in the same manner is able to correct its distortions. Its impact on the other fundamental aspect of vital energy is a little harder to show in a laboratory experiment. Time doesn't allow itself to be caught that easily.

Yet this feat may also be possible. I will tell you a short story that may tempt some inventive spirit to try the experiment. In the spring of 1982 I decided that, to minimize all the paperwork, this modern plague of our profession, I would computerize my office. With the help of a knowledgeable acquaintance I chose both machine and program. But owing to lack of space I was forced to install the equipment on a counter in my small laboratory. I don't think I have ever been as upset and nervous as during the 8 weeks following this change.

The start-up and apprenticeship of the programme proceeded smoothly until the machine suddenly began to have a series of breakdowns. I finally managed to prove to the repair engineer that my own skills (or lack thereof) weren't the cause of the difficulty, but he remained unable to find the reason for the mysterious malfunctions. One after the other, the various pieces and finally entire systems were replaced, but with no greater success. But more frustrating than anything else was the fact that the computer that the engineer had removed to his workshop remained 'sick' for a few days and then spontaneously 'recovered'. Meanwhile my new computer continued to break down, and one day in exasperation I asked the engineer to take it apart in front of me. To his amazement I proceeded to examine the machine with my pendulum and quickly located the source of our problems – an interface board about as big as a playing card, covered with microprocessors and containing a magnetic memory system. We replaced the defective part, and sure enough the computer once again worked. Immediately upon returning to his workshop the engineer retried the defective piece and found that it still malfunctioned. This remained true for the next few days until another spontaneous 'recovery' occurred and the part once again worked!

It was this impact of the time element on the state of my computer that provided me with a clue to the real source of the problem. It suddenly occurred to me that the machine had probably been contaminated by the emanations from the homoeopathic doses that I prepared daily in my laboratory. The machine was in fact installed on my very small workspace and its magnetic elements weren't protected from the rays of the high dilutions. In my experiments with the pendulum I had already noticed the impact they were able to exercise on gravitational fields when nearby. You may think that my imagination was running away with me but subsequent events were to prove me right. I moved the machine into the next room and have never had a breakdown since.

This story would seem to indicate that an experimental method could be developed to test the temporal effect of homoeopathic doses. I will happily contribute a few other suggestions to any serious team of researchers who would like to repeat my experience and try to capture a piece of time.

As for a scientific explanation of this phenomenon, I'm afraid my knowledge of experimental physics is too limited to allow a convincing explanation. However, from a superficial study of Feynman's diagrams showing the creation by a photon of the electron–positron couple, I have developed a hypothesis which I believe deserves the attention of physicists. For Richard Feynman, the positron is an electron that moves backward through time; in his zig-zagging spatiotemporal diagrams one sees how the electron is moved towards the past. One could almost say that it is programmed backwards. For me, there is an immediate analogy here with the homoeopathic dose, which I suspect might be discreetly emitting some kind of positrons (or antipositrons).

To support this hypothesis, an analysis of the fabrication process itself should be undertaken using the means of modern physics. You will remember that Hahnemann always insisted strongly on the absolute necessity of an 'elasticity' in the shock imparted in his process of dilution–potentization. In 1974, while reading the now famous work of S Ostrander and L Schroeder on the Russian studies in parapsychology, I was very impressed by the work of the astrophysicist Nicolai Kozyrev concerning the nature of time. One of the techniques he had imagined, to reveal the energy of time, was precisely the mechanical transcription of the temporal density of an elastic system under tension. In this way the density of time would become measurable. I am convinced that Hahnemann discovered in his elastic shock the simplest and most elegant way to achieve the required 'thickening' of temporal energy, a kind of 'compacting' of time.

Am I on the right track? Will it be possible one day to verify my hypotheses? And who could do so? I only know for certain that it will not be the doctors, since the scientific preparation that the future stars of our profession still receive today stops where it should start: it brings them only to the doorstep of the world of biophysics.

But luckily there is no need to wait for the endorsement of science to be able to act. The suffering of mankind is such that doctors not only have a right, but also a moral obligation, to use all the resources available to their intelligence in the attempt to heal. The immense majority of my colleagues are still satisfied with the ambiguous feats conferred by chemotherapy. I prefer using the wonderful possibilities contained in my nice little positron bombs. They have given me back the joy of healing, the secular vocation that is a very part of me.

In the following pages I will describe in more detail than is possible during a consultation the method that I have developed and untiringly explain at each first meeting with my patients. I have called it 'sequential therapy' because of its constant reference to the element of time. It is not perfect, nor a cure-all, but it has filled me with joy for many years. It is the first pillar of Real Medicine.

NINE

Sequential therapy

A young mother is sitting across from me with a child in her lap who is trying alternately to escape her discreet surveillance, or to be comforted by her. She is recounting her trials and tribulations, so common and distressing that as often happens when I listen to my patients I feel anger and revolt rising in me.

Regardless of the illness undermining the child's health, the story is always the same. After a few months of problem-free life, or sometimes almost immediately following the child's birth, motherhood has become an endless series of visits to the paediatrician and the pharmacy, anxiously awaiting the next day's events. At each visit there is a new prescription for an antibiotic, a sedative syrup, or an anti-inflammatory pill. In answer to questions about the real cause of the problem there are only evasive replies. Recovery seems indefinitely postponed, confidence diminishes and other specialists are visited. All in vain.

This frustrating trial of patience can last for years. In fact, it lasts just as long as the image of modern medicine continues to influence parents impressed by the breathtaking achievements of the men in white, held in such high esteem by our technologically oriented society, until finally the day comes when faced with such manifest and repeated failures, the mirage of 'easy' health dissipates. Anguished self-questioning then ensues. What if all the promises of medicine were only a bad joke? What if the immense technohospital machine was nothing but false security? It is only then, alas often late in the day, that, through chance conversations or information gleaned here and there, parents realize or remember that there are other ways – so-called 'alternative' ways – more gentle and more efficient in the long struggle to regain health.

It is in like manner that thousands of patients every year swell the ranks of homoeopathy. Some are disappointed and quickly return to their chemotherapists, but most remain. Ten years ago this trend was barely evident, but its growing size augurs well for the future. The only obstacle to an irresistible wave is the compartmentalized nature of current homoeopathic practice. There are almost as many techniques as there are homoeopaths! It is my dearest wish that this book contribute to the breaking down of barriers and to a more unified therapeutic approach.

I always impart the same information to a new patient, be it a young mother seeing me for the first time, a desperate and disillusioned patient trying his last chance or simply someone dissatisfied with another homoeopath's treatment. As it is not something I learned from books or copied from Hahnemann or other later masters, I take full responsibility for it. Here it is.

The entire art of healing is based on one unchanging principle: vital energy. Life is an unfolding of this vital energy. This is the fundamental principle of Real Medicine, the first commandment if you like. So from the very start the 'in-house' disagreement is self-evident as official medicine doesn't even recognize the existence of vital energy because it can't be measured. I freely admit that this is the case. But the fact that it is not possible as yet to measure it with our present instruments is not a good enough reason to deny its existence. It may be elusive, but it is none the less essential to life. All that one can say is that our techniques are not yet up to the challenge. Perhaps one day they will be, but for the moment we must be satisfied with an act of faith. Depending on whether a doctor chooses to make this act of faith or not, he opts for one or the other camp. It is in this manner that the dispute between these two forms of medicine often resembles the ferocity of a religious war. If you can accept this principle, this first step, then the entire art of healing is child's play since one obvious conclusion leads on to the next.

The second principle, following immediately from the first, cannot in any way be disputed rationally. Here it is not a question of an act of faith, but of mathematical reasoning. This second truth is as follows: all energy, no matter how noble, is governed by the law of bipolarity. All energy is by definition bipolar. This means that vital energy, like electrical energy for example, is by its very nature diphasic, defined by its positive and negative poles. This is merely the repetition of what the Chinese have known for centuries. The ancient wise men of Imperial China maintained that life was nothing more than energy (called Qi or Chi) and was defined by the intriguing alternation of Yin and Yang. At this moment in my presentation, I always point to the electrical cord of my desk lamp because today even children know that with only one wire the electrical current wouldn't produce light.

And from here the third principle can be expressed thus: life, like the electrical current travelling over the wires, is a fluid circulating freely back and forth in its alternating phases. Life isn't a static entity, it is a current which passes. And health, like the pleasant light from the bulb, is inconceivable without the balanced harmony of its positive and negative phases.

This extremely simplified reasoning allows us to understand the real nature of illness. Man falls ill because his vital energy no longer flows harmoniously in the dynamic balance of Yin and Yang, but instead moves like the flickering light from a partially unscrewed bulb or an overloaded circuit on a stormy evening. Illness is a breakdown in harmony, a distortion, a disorientation.

Given this, and faced with a clinical picture of impaired health (no matter what the current diagnosis may be), the one and only important question the doctor must pose to himself is this: why is the patient's vital energy out of phase?

This question, which is really **the** question, is precisely the one that doctors unfortunately never ask since they don't believe in vital energy! Which is why medical research fails so abysmally. Millions are spent and thousands of researchers are at work in all kinds of 'scientific' fields. But the one logical path is scrupulously avoided. This is the tragedy of present-day medicine leading to the disillusionment of the innumerable patients it cannot heal.

This colossal misunderstanding disappears once the true 'energy' nature of health is grasped. And a clear and precise answer can be given to the essential question posed above. In illness, vital energy is out of phase because it has been the victim of an aggression and is now twisted, distorted and imbalanced. It is like the interference in a badly tuned station on your radio, and health cannot be recovered until the balance is re-established much in the same way as one would adjust a dial on the radio or properly screw in a light bulb.

Illness is thus disharmony, the disruption of balance. What should the doctor do? To my mind, his most urgent task is to find the troublemaker, the cause of this imbalance. The guilty party is necessarily a disrupting shock, a parasite wavelength upsetting the vital energy's harmonious movement. Its nature can be as diverse as the multiple facets of material reality, since everything that exists in the universe is energy, and any event is by definition an unfolding of energy. If the event is harmonious, in phase with our vital energy, health is conserved. If the parasite wavelength makes its presence felt at the wrong time a struggle ensues, there is violent confrontation, and derailment occurs. The Chinese quite rightly speak of 'perverse' energies. Indeed, illness is the perversion of our energetic balance.

If you take the time to examine your own life, you will likely be in agreement with the following reasoning. From birth our organism is subjected to the many energetic confrontations of existence. Our body, a wonderfully complex system, is constantly subjected to the energetic variations of our environment. We are subject to the alternation of day and night, to variations in atmospheric pressure and composition, to assaults from unknown cosmic forces, to seasons, storms, drought, and to the implacable sun. And yet we don't fall ill from these things; we adapt. In winter we are cold, in summer, the heat tires us, but our corrective mechanisms prevent a catastrophic deregulation of our energetic commands. Quite simply, the powerful flux of our vital energy is not thrown off balance by such trifles.

The same is true of the many events that occur during our lives: the small dissatisfactions and anxieties, the minor cuts and bruises, accidents and illnesses, the inevitable occasionally hurt feelings. Popular wisdom has noticed that a good dose of the flu treated at home, lasts from 7 to 15 days ... or two weeks if the doctor intervenes! Our vital energy is strong enough to cope with most of these disruptions. It is momentarily imbalanced, depending on the violence of the shock, then it continues its majestic course, like a great river only slightly and superficially troubled by the sudden influx of a violent mountain stream.

Most illnesses spontaneously heal in this way provided two conditions are met. First of all, the vital current must be strong. If the mountain torrent is stronger than the weak river in the plain, it is the torrent that will impose its law as soon as they meet. A robust young man stuck in bed with a case of broncho-pneumonia can overcome without too much trouble the morbid shock, but not so a tired old man or an immature baby.

The other condition is the time factor. The twisted energy will regain its balance again, provided the disturbance doesn't continue for too long. A life in which nothing occurs is like the calm mirror of a pond's surface. The stone that a passer-by throws into the water creates a rippling disturbance, which gradually disappears with time, even if the stone is large. If your vital energy is thrown out of phase by a bad case of viral hepatitis, it will still recover provided you undertake the indispensable long rest of a perhaps boring convalescence. You will then be ready to deal with the next set of events.

The essential thing to recognize is that our lives are a long succession of more or less violent energetic interferences, which trouble the harmonious flow of our vital energy. Luckily, big shocks are less frequent than small ones and there are also long periods of calm. This alternation of disturbances and repose explains the relative rarity of serious illness. Between bouts there is enough time for our vitality to be restored.

But life is unfortunately not always so generous. For some, the intense shocks are really too difficult to overcome. For others, those who seem jinxed, the continuous succession of shocks is so confusing that their vital energy can never regain control of the situation. And serious or chronic illness creeps into their lives, remaining mysterious or disconcerting for those who have been unable to come to terms with the weight of these successive events.

Now we all know that everything has its price; each abrupt gesture takes its toll and each wound leaves a mark. Any shock will leave a trace, large or small, depending on the violence of the impact, visible and palpable if the surface is material, invisible but none the less present when the surface is immaterial. If the shocks are repeated, the material surface receiving them will become scratched and bumpy. The same result occurs from the shocks hammering at our vital fibre even if the consequences escape our attention at the time.

'Show us these marks!', the more 'scientific' minds will say, 'we want to touch them with our hands.' We admit that there are sequels to polio, and that smallpox scars, but why the devil invoke 'immaterial traces?'. Of course, you are right, dear, sceptical colleague, I cannot point them out with my finger. Here, as we saw earlier about vital energy, it is only through faith, or perhaps a real scientific spirit, that this hypothesis can be accepted. I accepted it ... and have had the immense joy of being able to verify it too.

My brand-new experience with the Vollian techniques that I had learned in Lausanne had opened my eyes to the immaterial reality of the Chinese meridians. Like all adepts of this method I was able to see the obvious disturbances in the electrical permeability of chronically ill patients. Like them, I was able to identify with the ohmmeter certain homoeopathic nosodes that seemed capable of re-establishing the lost harmony. But very quickly, starting in 1975, I came up against the first experimental contradictions. After a phase of disappointment, I finally understood the reason. Voll's technique concerns the meridians, but the measurements take place on the physical body at the meeting point of the immaterial meridian and the material support. The point tested is like a bridge, a kind of soldered joint. My limited knowledge of oriental medicine suggested that by only testing the nosodes on the material surface I was making the same mistake as a purchaser of a black and white television who is surprised at not seeing images in colour.

Voll's technique leads one to draw conclusions concerning the quality of the transmission when in fact it can only reveal the parameters of reception. The ohmmeter makes no distinction between the transmitting point and the receiving terminal. Now everybody should know that our physical body is merely the most material of the vehicles for our soul. The vital energy that animates it passes through several successive layers of vibration that are fully recognized by oriental philosophy and medicine before becoming denser in the complex network of the Chinese meridians, the last prematerial stage of the downward movement of divine energy. By testing the quality of vibrations sensed by the receiver, one obviously cannot judge the quality or flaws of the transmission. How can one judge the quality of a Beethoven symphony by hearing it transmitted on a cheap portable radio?

In diagnosing an illness normal doctors consider only the material causes, those which mark the physical body. With Voll's method it is more or less possible to refine the investigation by taking it to the limit between the physical shell and the first energetic envelope. All that is needed is the ohmmeter. But already at this stage the doctor's personality plays a major role since it is not really possible to separate oneself from the different energetic envelopes whose essential property is to vibrate.

The doctor's vibrations will naturally interfere with those of the patient. (I hope that this will help you to understand the curious events described in Chapter 6.) This is also the reason why it is important to choose an optimistic and healthy doctor. If the doctor has a powerful vital 'radiation', his high-frequency energy will inevitably help the weaker energy of his patient. The ohmmetric test will be skewed and everything will seem vibrationally as being in order. To discover the morbid disharmony the examination must take place at the level of the energetic envelope, which is often called the 'astral body', and not at the the soldered points of the frontier one level down, which is called the 'etheric body'.

The working level and the vibrational frequency of the examination must thus be raised. Unfortunately there are few doctors capable of this. And before anything else can be done they have to recognize the necessity of doing so! The only practitioners who even accept the principle are homoeopaths and acupuncturists, and most of these use only tried and proven techniques or the artifices of modern technology. This is true despite the fact (as I hope I have helped you to understand in my chapter on vital energy) that the only way to reach the higher spheres is to raise one's own consciousness until what might be called a state of grace (commonly called a 'gift') has been achieved. Some reach this level through suffering, others through meditation or other spiritual exercises.

The acquisition of this new sensitivity is never easy. In my case, the 12 years of experimentation with radiesthesia were the price that I had to pay to achieve this state of grace. I understood this clearly the day that I was testing an 'incriminated' nosode in the hand of one of my patients, and at the same moment that I unblocked one of the two key meridians, the pendulum's movement was inversed. The patient very clearly felt a small electrical charge all along the meridian. Following this first revelation in 1975, this phenomenon repeated itself thousands of times and allowed me to develop progressively a radiesthesic technique that I may one day publish.

But a description of technical methods is not the objective of this book. I just want to emphasize that it is possible to find all the events that have marked our energetic systems. Whether with a pendulum or any other superior sensory mechanism, success will come only to those who have been able to elevate the level at which they are working. And, even so, they have to be willing to work at it. 'Only he who seeks shall find!' That person alone will experience the joy of discovering the surprisingly rich energetic network of our lives in all its strengths and weaknesses.

Starting in 1975 I began a real detective's investigation with my patients, seeking all the events of their lives that could possibly have left immaterial traces. I became an archaeologist of the astral body, examining every scar and bump on their invisible shells. And what I found amazed me! While Voll's machine had permitted certain discoveries, my new technique revealed every thread and knot. I quickly had to accept that the list of events that leave an indelible mark on our energetic cloak is far longer than might be expected. If anything it resembles the long list of intuitive worries of a young mother watching for every possible threat to her child. The following is a classical repertory of these inevitable shocks which modulate our lives.

Already at birth there are plenty of opportunities to lose our wonderful Yin and Yang balance: prolonged or artificially shortened labour, forceps and other instruments, lengthy periods of cerebral anoxia, operation in the case of Caesarean birth, insufficient or asymmetrical modelling of the skull. I will mention later some methods to correct the traces of these first accidents.

And then almost immediately and always too soon – while the infant is still in its cot – the modern paediatrician will perpetrate what nature in all its wisdom would never allow to occur. Without batting an eyelid he inflicts a series of intense energetic shocks on the poor young creature from which some will never recover. You will never see your children fall ill on the same day with measles, mumps and chicken-pox. Nature isn't cruel enough to do such a thing. If by chance your child comes down with the measles while just recovering from scarlet fever you will remember for many a year that dreadful period and your poor child's suffering. Yet your paediatrician sincerely believes that he is helping your child's chances of survival by inoculating him on the same day against four illnesses, at least three of which are potentially fatal! Unquestionably the discovery of vaccinations was a great step forward for our civilization, but it never should have engendered the current waste that is responsible for so many hidden deaths and innumerable chronic illnesses. Vaccinate against diphtheria, tetanus and polio – yes, by all means. But why all on the same day? Why so early? Why so abruptly with no preparation for the shock? Every vaccination, even the ridiculous (and not very efficient) whooping cough vaccination that so many doctors insist on adding to the three others, is without exception a shock.

And if the homoeopathic experience has shown that the first vaccination is capable of leaving an indelible mark, imagine what further imbalance is created by each booster shot that is intended to increase and strengthen the immunity. These repetitions can sometimes create such confusion that the delicate health of certain children is definitively compromised. And then the chemical warfare begins, the onslaught of increasingly 'deadly' chemical weapons under the orders of the person in the white coat. What this all-powerful person does not know is that there are other more efficient ways to solidly and definitively reinforce immunity. I will go into these in detail in the next part of this book. For the moment you should simply remember that every vaccination marks for ever the core of the 70,000 billion cells of our physical body. It is certainly hard to imagine a worse shock!

Another key period of our lives, and one full of destabilizing events, is early childhood. It is the critical period involving the childhood illnesses that marks us every bit as much as the vaccinations mentioned above. The daily practice of homoeopathy has also taught me (and other homoeopathic doctors as well) that a shock can come from any event and at any age – for example a sudden and strong fright, an immense sadness or disappointment, an operation or even a common concussion. One must also include such events as a major haemorrhage, a blood transfusion or an abortion, any prolonged chemotherapy, particularly antibiotic and antidepressive, or use of the drug cortisone. Drug addicts and alcoholics are of course constantly being shocked.

And then there are the serious illnesses, which can easily be understood as being disruptive to energetic balance. I am not speaking here of banal sore throats, earaches, bronchitis, etc, but of specific diseases caused by recognized agents and which create a clearly defined clinical picture. For example syphilis, malaria or tuberculosis. A primary tubercular infection or a case of typhoid fever is never inoffensive. Toxoplasmosis can be a terrible shock, as can brucellosis, leptospirosis, viral hepatitis and so on.

You see that the list is already long, and yet I will add to it shortly. But the important thing to retain here, the really interesting fact, is the enormous disparity between the energetic consequences of these events. Some seem to inflict an enormous shock and in fact leave almost no trace. Others that are apparently insignificant leave after-effects that can destroy an entire life. Their relative importance is very unequal. This is certainly due to the multiplicity of paths taken by vital energy and the numerous intricacies resulting from the different shocks.

The chronology of events is also important. The overall energetic picture won't be the same if the successive shocks deforming the energetic ribbon have done so in one sequence rather than another. Your child's health won't be the same when he is 10 if he had German measles at age 3, measles at 7 and mumps at 9 instead of measles at age 3, mumps at 7 and German measles at 9. In the first case his health will be better since the events occurred in the classical order designed by nature. But even then, if the measles at age 7 didn't go well, perhaps owing to a bad case of flu just before, this judgement could easily be wrong.

As you can easily imagine, the doctor's art is really the unravelling of the subtle fabric of influences making up our lives. He must spot each suspect occurrence, identify the guilty parties and establish a clear chronology of events. In essence, this fascinating work of energetic diagnosis is really a disentangling of a momentarily confused spatiotemporal skein through finding the sequence of large and small events that have created the knots. This is diagnosis deserving of the name, the only truly useful preliminary work because it reveals the real causes of illness.

Once the cause is identified, treatment becomes possible. And the proposed treatment is completely logical. Since the illness comes from an imbalance, the treatment must re-establish that balance. Since the illness comes from a series of disturbing shocks that are characterized by a series of traces, the treatment must erase these traces in the same sequential order, but backwards. And how does one erase the trace of a shock? By repeating the same shock of course, but in the opposite direction.

I always compare my work to that of a panel-beater. A brush is not going to be enough to remove the dents from a car's surface. First they will have to be hammered out from beneath with an equal strength to the initial accidental shock. This is what I do with my patients. I erase the deformations of their astral bodies. But there is an additional difficulty in my work. The panel-beater can smooth out all the dents at one time since his work area has only the three dimensions of space while my hammering involves a fourth dimension, our old friend time. I can't smooth out in one go the rough angles of childhood, the savage upheavals of puberty and the powerful surges of adulthood. Don't ever forget this: our successive energetic layers contain all four dimensions of the space–time continuum!

The logical treatment must therefore be a volley of blows. Very specifically, a minutely orchestrated sequence of equalizing shocks. There is no need for concern since I won't be using the big club of modern chemotherapy in my attack. How could I, since the correction must be administered going backwards through time? The only means at my disposition capable of removing the destructive scars of the past will come from homoeopathy. (Acupuncture could also claim similar powers, but with far more difficulty and with no guarantee of lasting success.) No other medical technique can offer such elegance and efficiency. No other technique is as close as this to the immateriality of life because a homoeopathic remedy is not an ordinary material substance. It is neither vegetable, mineral nor chemical in nature. It is immaterial energy precisely because it is created by the elimination of material substance.

You will remember my definition of a homoeopathic remedy. I explained that a correctly potentized dose is like a small time-machine. For each important event in my patient's life I look for the closest, the 'most similar' homoeopathic remedy, which is able to imprint an identical destabilizing wave on the disturbed energetic balance. And then, blow by blow, I re-establish the balance no matter how long ago the shock took place. This is because I can do more than choose the target; I can also adjust the potency and the exact distance of the shot. All I have to do is adjust the time-clock on my delayed-reaction bomb. If the retrogressive explosion coincides exactly with that of the old shock then I have succeeded: bull's-eye!

If the ammunition that I use is of the same nature as the event that caused the problem, then the equalizing shock is nearly perfect. This is isopathy, and the 'bomb' is a nosode. For example, in order to annihilate the nasty immaterial distortion left by scarlet fever, the nosode Scarlatinum is perfect. It is actually prepared from a culture of the haemolytic streptococcus that causes the illness, but is rendered inoffensive by the dematerialization resulting from the dilution–potentization process.

If the remedy used is not of the same nature as the imbalance being attacked, the equalizing shock will not be as perfect, but none the less very efficient. We are talking here about homoeopathy. The 'bomb' is the simillimum. To erase the traces of an old cerebral concussion, the simillimum Natrium sulphuricum will be perfect since this is what the 'portrait' of an intoxication from sodium sulphate most resembles.

I am sure that you have noticed that I often use the word 'shock'. This is intentional. It is essential to recognize that this sequential treatment is not harmless. It really is a serious energetic bombardment and it would be wrong to minimize its effects on the overall condition of the patient. Only children seem to be able to bear up easily under this treatment since they have tremendous energetic resources. Most adults are exhausted by the treatment or have unpleasant reactions, particularly on the days when the 'bomb' finds its target.

It is also important to mention that women should not take nosodes or any other isopathics during their menstrual periods because they would risk passing some disagreeable days and their cycle could be disturbed. I also interrupt the sequential treatment during the first 3 months of a pregnancy, not because of any risk to the child or mother, but in order to avoid increased fatigue during this critical period.

* * *

In summarizing the essential elements of this long theoretical introduction, I must emphasize strongly that illness is fundamentally energetic. Life is the flow of vital energy and is bipolar and divine. When the flow is harmonious, health is guaranteed. If the harmony is broken, no matter at what level, illness will follow. To re-establish health, the doctor must identify the disturbing elements and neutralize them. He (or she) does have the means to do this, the absolute weapon – the homoeopathic remedy, a tiny package of immaterial energy, a fragment of space and time. To each past event generating an instability, the doctor will oppose a specific quantum of energy, bit by bit freeing the vital energy, which is the prisoner of its own scars.

If the doctor is a clever detective, he will find the slightest suspect deviations and will be very successful. Less gifted, but conscientious in his work, he should try to establish the most detailed anamnesis that he can, strictly respecting the chronological sequence. From this point on he must act on the principle that every element is a likely suspect and if necessary must be homoeopathically erased. The resultant sequential treatment will be less elegant, but every bit as efficient.

Obviously this treatment is perfect for children. Their mother's memories are clear, their medical records have not yet been lost, vaccination records are precise and the memory of prior treatments is still very much alive. In Part II of this book, I will show how the sequential treatment (which in the ideal case is perfectly 'isosequential') frequently results in a spectacular cure of the innumerable illnesses that so often can make one doubt the perfection of creation.

But the method does more than correct the misfortunes of life. It achieves maximum efficiency when it reaches the area of prenatal history, the infamous predispositions, which are carried across the generations by our genetic code. This is where the homoeopathic remedy reveals its truly fantastic abilities and seems capable of the impossible.

But before talking about the full possibilities of the integral treatment in its entirety – which is the subject of Part III – we will review the many occasions where it is not necessary to go that far to obtain a bountiful harvest.

PART TWO

PRACTICE
Healing through homoeopathic sequential therapy

TEN

Childhood ailments

This chapter presents the reader with a patchwork of the common ailments that relentlessly pursue certain children, returning again and again as the weeks and months go by. I am speaking here of the innumerable flus, chronic bronchitis and sinusitis that go on and on, reappearing with the slightest draft of cold air. Or it can be sore throats and/or earache with sudden crises of fever and violent pain. The nights are long and punctuated by the child's crying and discomfort; relapses occur without warning, in summer as in winter; grandmothers complain that there are no longer any normal seasons.

After a few years of this purgatory these 'minor ailments' become intolerable, and mothers become seriously worried. Why can't the paediatrician find the right treatment? What is being hidden from me? And what if my child isn't normal? Sometimes the parents' concern turns to anguish as the diminishing resistance of their children becomes so critical that survival seems totally dependent on the consumption of increasingly stronger antibiotics. I encounter these despairing and disappointed parents every week, and I often hear the same disillusioned remark: 'What's the point of going back to the paediatrician? All he'll do is prescribe another antibiotic that won't work any better than the last one. Too bad you can't buy them at the supermarket. We could manage without a doctor!'

Unfortunately this is a sad reality of our times. Every day, medicine is losing its devotees by the thousand, since millions of people across the world are noticing doctors' complete incompetence when faced with these common problems. In fact one couldn't imagine a more banal situation. This mountain of small human miseries is the direct result of a very ordinary energetic imbroglio which the doctors have at least partly created themselves. Yes, it is possible to state that almost all of these problems are iatrogenic – in plain English this means caused by the medicine. A few examples will make this clearer.

Case 1.

I had a visit in March 1981 from Benoît D, born in 1977 in the Valais (one of the Swiss cantons). At the age of 4 months he had a serious case of bronchitis and was treated with Clamoxyl, a popular antibiotic. This vigorous treatment didn't improve his health, quite the contrary, since his general condition deteriorated rapidly and catastrophically. The bouts of bronchitis followed each other relentlessly and became complicated by a false croup. From his 5th to his 24th month the child was 'fed on Clamoxyl' (his mother's expression), and to no avail. The paediatrician decided on hospitalization and the identical treatment continued in the hospital. After all, why change? Isn't this antibiotic therapy the summum of the healing art? Shortly following his return home the first relapse occured – more bronchitis and blow after blow of the medical hammer. At 2½ years, the child was a mere shadow and couldn't tolerate anything. A decision to operate (something had to be done!) was taken and the specialist removed the adenoids. The bronchitis stopped, but not the colds, which became more and more severe with high fever and extreme fatigue. Naturally the paediatrician intervened brilliantly each time with his Clamoxyl. But nature has its limits, even for this robust little boy.

His white blood cell counts began to lack. The inspired paediatrician decided to swap hammers and prescribed Bactrim. There was no reaction and the child was admitted to intensive care from which he emerged 15 days later, out of danger, but still not cured. Bronchitis then reappeared, Clamoxyl was administered at each new alert, freeing the doctor from his medical responsibility but the child that I then had before me was no longer a child. It was a poor silent thing, a shadow, a caricature. What would his future life be? The parents anxiously awaited each relapse and the white cell count stubbornly refused to improve.

What could I do for this little boy? The answer is easy. I quite simply changed his destiny by doing my normal work as a doctor. First the diagnosis: it leaps out at you. The boy was suffering from an enormous imbalance in his vital energy. Why? Because the imbalance had been created. By what? By the following disturbing sequence of events: BCG (tuberculosis) vaccination at birth – severe bronchitis at 4 months – Clamoxyl – DiTePerPol vaccination (diphtheria, tetanus, whooping cough and polio) vaccination – Clamoxyl – booster DTPP – Clamoxyl – DTPP – Clamoxyl – Clamoxyl – Clamoxyl – Clamoxyl – Clamoxyl – surgical operation – Bactrim – mumps – measles vaccination – Clamoxyl – Clamoxyl – Clamoxyl ... And in all this series the only shock that occurred naturally was the mumps. Everything else was iatrogenic. How could I re-establish the balance? By erasing the immaterial traces of these shocks one at a time, following the reverse chronological order.

First I removed the traces of the antibiotics and the surgical operation with isotherapy and the appropriate homoeopathic remedies. The reaction was a severe cold. In April I erased the artificial measles with the measles nosode called Morbillinum. The reaction was a temperature of 104°F and a face as red as a beetroot. At the end of May I removed the ghost of the mumps with the nosode Parotidinum and in mid July, the four DTPP vaccinations with their respective nosodes. At the end of August I dealt the final blow with the nosode for the terrible BCG vaccination, which was probably the cause of the entire disaster in the first place.

I saw the child again in September. A miracle had taken place! He had regained a healthy complexion and was at last eating; he had a more expansive character and his little friends allowed him to play with them. His vital energy was back on a harmonious course. He was cured! I saw him three more times over the following year to fortify his basic constitution, and he has not been seriously ill since then. His three brothers went through the same treatment to remove the same iatrogenic problems as his and here we now have a whole family that won't be easily fooled again by the allopathic doctors and their chemicals.

Case 2.

On 6 July 1983 I received Diane G from Geneva, aged 6 months. Her parents had come to me because they felt that the child had been unable to recover from her first DTPP vaccination. It seemed that shortly following this first shock she had developed a slight fever which failed to disappear. The child had ceased to be cheerful, and the parents to have peace of mind. It is difficult not to imagine the worst with a sickly child who has run a fever for 3 months. The paediatrician claimed that it had nothing to do with the vaccination and after examining the child declared this to be a slight cold and (as he was taught by the faculty) reasoned that since there was a fever there must be an inflammation which would have to be treated with an anti-inflammatory drug. A great idea, was it not? The doctor prescribed Tylenol (a popular drug containing paracetamol, a fairly common and toxic substance used in many children's suppositories). Unfortunately the fever refused to go away. Worse, the baby's cheerful character disappeared completely, and the parents lost all confidence in their doctor. They could hardly be blamed since the doctor had managed to mis-diagnose the problem totally. The parents – the non-specialists – were absolutely right and the specialist absolutely wrong! The only illness involved here was the distortion of vital energy resulting from the hammer blows of the vaccination.

The appropriate treatment was immediately decided. I mixed the four DTPP nosodes and administered them immediately. Five days later the father called to confirm the fever's disappearance and a spectacular improvement in the child's overall condition. Over the next 10 months there were four more visits to strengthen the general constitution of this child who had now become a lovely and robust little girl. I can assure you that these parents aren't in any hurry to consult their doctor again

Case 3.

In January 1981 I saw Françoise H, from Carouge, Geneva. Born in 1968, this lovely young girl's life was plagued by a chronic cold which appeared to be resistant to all the treatments proposed by my learned colleagues. Her problems started very early – in

December 1968 immediately following a smallpox vaccination. Her mother told the following story: in December, first flu – in February 1969 a 102°F fever following the DTPP vaccination – and then the chronically present cold – in July 1969 a nasty virus still encountered some resistance and the resultant fever jumped to 104°F – the poor child wouldn't be this lucky in the future because the paediatrician decided to contribute to the existing imbalance by adding a measles vaccination in February 1970 – from here on everything went wrong, the cold became a spasmodic croup that managed to reappear four times despite the various treatments proposed – her adenoids were removed in the winter of 1970 with no results – the spasmodic croup reappeared and the adenoids grew back – a second operation took place a year later which resulted in a severe infection and transformed the cold into a chronic case of tracheitis – the spasmodic croup reappeared, and following a BCG vaccination, life became a constant string of colds and bronchitis.

Finally, a 'specialist' was consulted who performed allergy tests. The results were marvellous: the child was allergic to everything! One might have guessed as much! So the treatment was changed and the paediatrician prescribed Co-tylenol. This is made of paracetamol reinforced with two molecules that are every bit as toxic but are supposed to have an anti-allergenic effect. The result was pitiful, with secondary effects adding themselves to the primary reactions. But do you think the doctor would lay down his weapons? Not at all! He succeeded in exacerbating the existing disorder by vaccinating the same day for mumps and German measles. This was really the last straw; the parents finally realized that their daughter would never be cured in this way.

What was she suffering from? Now you too know the answer. The child's vital energy had been dramatically distorted by the unfortunately archiclassical iatrogenic sequence: vaccinations for smallpox – DTPP – DTPP – DTPP – DTPP – measles – BCG – German measles – mumps. My treatment respected this order and reversed its direction. I prescribed the following nosodes: Parotidinum – Rubeolinum – BCG – Morbillinum – DTPP – Vaccinotoxinum. This sequential treatment took 8 months and in September 1981 when I saw Françoise again she was transformed. There were still occasional colds, but without the complications. Each one of the shocks administered by my treatment had been very tiring, sometimes with uncomfortable reactions, but she had grown considerably and was again enjoying life. It took me 2 more years to correct the genetic flaw that was in fact the cause of all this misery, but today she is cured and 'vaccinated' for life against the excesses of 'normal' medicine, officialized by the faculty. Perhaps you think that this was a harmless case and that the child would have recovered spontaneously with the onset of puberty? You are perfectly at rights to think so, but it is certainly not the opinion of her mother. Unfortunately Françoise's mother knows the price that has to be paid for listening to the allopathic practitioners. Having followed their counsel this woman herself is now a chronic asthmatic completely dependent on the sinister drug, cortisone.

Case 4.

In January 1982 I saw a young child named Hervé T, from Neuchâtel. His history was simple. Born in August 1978, he was healthy until that autumn despite a slight heart murmur. His first shock was in October with the BCG vaccination, followed by DTPP in November, December and January. Problems started to show in the summer and the baby had 15 cases of throat inflammation over the following two years, all 'cut off' by Clamoxyl. The paediatrician also administered Ospen, which is just another name for penicillin. As a means of helping protect the little patient (remember he has a weak heart) a measles vaccination before the age of 2 years was administered. The same year the poor child came down with mumps and the attacks of throat inflammation continued unabated. Why? Because the doctor wasn't trying to find the cause of the problem. It's so much simpler just to follow the instructions from the faculty and keep to the role of salesman for the powerful drug companies. The tax payer forks out, and medical responsibility is covered.

At the 19th case of throat inflammation, the parents began to question events, but not the paediatrician. This was the reason for their visit to my office. You already know my diagnosis: an enormous iatrogenic distortion from the vaccinations and antibiotics. The treatment wasn't simple. The child was like a sponge full of penicillin. He responded to each of my sequential doses in the only language which his body knew: more throat inflammation. But I am not the lackey of the chemical industry and I got him back on to his feet with immaterial doses of mercury and oligo-elements.

Following the sequential treatment I saw him again in April 1982. He was then 3½ years and in top form! His recovery from the 23rd attack of throat inflammation, which corresponded to my last dose of the treatment, had passed off without difficulty. Most of the cleaning out had been accomplished with the doses of Parotidinum, Morbillinum, DTPP and BCG and the iatrogenic nightmare is now a thing of the past. It took fully another year to repair the genetic code responsible for both the weak heart and the ENT (ear, nose and throat) problem. As you might have guessed, even though it is just one more thing that doctors don't know, the predisposition for both is the same.

Case 5.

I saw Laurent E from the Valais for the first time in August 1983 at the age of 9 years. This time it wasn't colds or bronchitis that I was dealing with, but 2 years of repeated attacks of bronchopneumonia. The family doctor, the paediatrician and the hospital couldn't find the reason. How could they without knowing the energetic foundations of life? Their materialist treatments only added chemical pollution to the energy distortion. Laurent's case was quite serious; both major meridians were blocked and no electrical current passed. Two other key meridians, the Lungs and Large Intestine, were flawed. With such a young child this was a very serious sign. I began the treatment by erasing the iatrogenic intoxication of the antibiotics. The reaction was violent: an asthma crisis lasting 1 day and 2 nights and pointing directly to the underlying constitution. But this was no time to stir up his heredity with the powerful homoeopathic constitutional remedies. The sequential treatment required a strict respect of Hering's Law, so I proceeded with Varicellinum at the end of August for the recent case of chicken-pox and then Morbillinum (for the measles) at the beginning of October. On 8 November when I saw Laurent again, all the meridians were clear. His mother was amazed by the change that had taken place. Even the family doctor quite elegantly recognized the fact. I continued with DTPP in November and finally BCG in December. The reactions to each were strong, including the flu in January, which was probably the BCG reaction, but the meridians stayed free throughout and the energetic circuits functioned.

I saw the child again in March, and the success of my first therapeutic sequence was clear. It was Laurent's first winter without broncho-pneumonia. The work that remained was to correct the defective genetic base. I had already started that second bombardment in February with small adjustments in March and April. In May I saw the child once again and everyone agreed that his transformation was frankly miraculous. His grades in school had improved because he was no longer frequently absent. (When he was being treated chemically he spent long weeks at home each year.) The parents had recovered their peace of mind and entrusted me with the treatment of their other children.

Case 6.

Young Yvan M from Lausanne was born in 1978 and was healthy until the first DTPP vaccinations, which began at the age of 5 months. The iatrogenic pneumonia that followed rapidly degenerated and it became clear that the illness was turning into severe asthma. The paediatrician wanted to further his misdeed by the use of cortisone. Fortunately today's mothers have more sense than their doctors, and Mme M refused and went to see a homoeopath. He was quite successful in keeping the illness in abeyance by using the method called 'draining' and several nosodes appropriate to Yvan's basic constitution. But he didn't respect Hering's Law, and was acting directly on the spatial structures of the genetic code, forgetting that they also have a temporal dimension. If he had been taking care of the child since birth everything would have been fine, but the paediatrician had done his work and its imprint was now indelibly marked on the thread of life. These traces had to be erased before going even further back. As this wasn't done, the homoeopath was no longer in control of the situation, the child suffered continuous otitis and the wonderful immaterial remedies were without effect.

Since the mother had herself been treated by me for the

previous 2 years, she quickly understood the reasons for the failure. I first saw Yvan in April 1984. Quite naturally he had a major blockage of the 'Heart Governor' meridian. The corrective sequence was quickly readjusted to erase the most recent events: measles in February 1984, chicken-pox in January 1983 before finally getting to the DTPP of 1978. The frequency and severity of the otitis had by then diminished, to be eliminated entirely when I went further back in genetic time.

Case 7.

Young Mathias H from Lucerne was born in 1972 with a similar destiny, but his story was even more instructive. His birth was induced following a premature breaking of the waters. The delivering doctor, who was unaware of the subtleties of cranial osteopathy, neglected to remodel the skull, which had been deformed. This serious professional mistake, perpetrated daily in obstetric wards, was to have unforeseen consequences on the innervation of the eye and the normal flow of tears. At 3 months were the first vaccination shock, throat inflammation, antibiotics, etc. At 5 months, and in the midst of the iatrogenic imbalance created by successive booster shots, the child was given two successive general anaesthesias necessary for the eye operations. From this moment on his vital energy was totally dephased. He no longer played, was sad and apathetic and his slow mental development was fully apparent when at the age of 3 years he was still not talking. Evocations of the infant Einstein's famous mutism didn't keep his parents from worrying, particularly as the child's health deteriorated into a never-ending series of feverish states and repeated attacks of throat inflammation. You can imagine the treatment: antibiotics, anti-inflammatory drugs, antibiotics, anti-inflammatories, etc. Then came the first neurological signs and an impairment of the lower limbs. At this point the worries had turned to outright anguish. The erudite colleagues murmured quietly the dreadful diagnosis: the child was spastic!

Luckily the parents no longer fully trusted their allopathic doctors and sought advice from a colleague who had taken the trouble to complete his medical studies at Dr Senn's school. Some hope returned when a small measure of vital energy was still found and they started a treatment that was to last 2 years. Unfortunately, the child made no progress at all. Disappointed, but intelligent, the parents didn't incriminate homoeopathy and found their way to my office. From the first ohmmetric reading I could see what had been wrong. The electrical current passed freely on all the meridians as if nothing were wrong at all! This was a classic stumbling-block of Voll's technique. Clearly the severity of the iatrogenic attack had atrociously mutilated the child's astral body. I started my sequential bombardment as follows: Morbillinum in October 1981, BCG in mid November and Varicellinum at the end of December.

In January, when I saw the child again, his father was fascinated and full of thanks. The boy was transformed: more active, and less introverted. I continued the treatment with Rubeolinum in February, Penicillinum in March and Parotidinum in the beginning of April. At the end of April in my office Mathias was not just transformed, but transfigured! He spoke, acted his age, and, although still timid, had become sociable. I gave him a dose of Pulsatilla, the classical remedy for timidity that the colleague preceding me had tried in vain. This time the effect was spectacular, and I brought my sequential treatment to a close with the DTPP bomb whose explosion was adjusted for the year 1972. The effect was overwhelming. The father spoke of a resurrection! When the child returned in September he was lively, cheerful, had stopped dragging his leg and was doing extremely well in school. Not bad for someone who was supposedly severely mentally handicapped! Of course, according to the wise men to whom our government has entrusted the teaching of medicine I have achieved these results strictly through the placebo effect!

* * *

I could continue with cases like these for hours, and had in fact selected a whole pile of files from my archives that are at least as evocative. But the repetition of the same facts quickly becomes tiresome. I think you have now understood how ill 'official' medicine really is and how badly in need of renovation.

I will leave the closing words of this chapter to a charming mother, straight from the country, who came to my office in April 1984 to introduce me to her two little girls, Marlène and Céline.

I asked her the reason of her visit, and she replied that she just wanted to meet me so as to have a real doctor at hand in the improbable case that her two daughters fall ill. Surprised I asked, 'They've never been ill?' To which she immediately and confidently answered, 'Oh no, why should they have been? They've never been to see a doctor!'

ELEVEN

Overvaccination and pervaccination

It is clear that the discovery of microbial agents marked a decisive turning point in the history of medicine. No one contests this and doctors cannot help but being delighted. It is, however, just as certain that this discovery has led the practice of healing into the dangerous waters of easy solutions and that its direct corollary has been the impoverishment of causal reasoning, which alone is capable of establishing the truth.

Reflection and experience irrefutably prove that the germ is not the primary cause of illness. The prior collapse of the body's defence systems clearly overshadows the importance of the role of germs, which more often is one of an impetus to or even merely a consequence of illness. It is my profound conviction that the germ conquers only when our organism allows it to do so. This is the true primary condition of all illness. Infectious agents can multiply and prosper only in a weakened terrain that has been devitalized by the lamentable disharmony of its vital energy.

The analogy with the art of war is striking: the enemy's attack succeeds only where the frontier is badly defended. If the fortification is strong enough there can be no victory for the intruder. If the attacked population is not united, or is poorly governed by useless leaders, the harmony of the social body is compromised and political stability has disappeared. Then the attacking hordes will spread like an epidemic unleashed by some mysterious signal that neither strategists nor doctors will be able to identify with certitude.

I am also convinced that the intimate mechanisms of epidemics have not yet been explicitly clarified and that viruses and microbes are just the first to benefit from the subterranean disharmony introduced by a common occult cause. It certainly appears that specific illnesses are caused by the invasion of certain specific germs. The treponema *T. pallidum* provokes genital chancres and Koch's bacillus tuberculizes the tissues, but they in themselves cannot cause syphilis or tuberculosis. For the illness to take hold, the terrain must first allow it to; the defensive systems must give way!

This notion was fully recognized by the first vaccinator of the Western world, a prudent English gentleman-farmer who had the courage to inoculate himself with the eruptive disease of cattle (cowpox) to protect himself from the dreadful effects of smallpox, one of the great scourges of his period. It was Lady Montague who really launched the practice by inoculating her own son in 1717. The principle was taken up again at the end of the same century by the well-known doctor named Edward Jenner, who codified the process and gave it the name 'vaccination'. These precursors unconsciously followed a truly homoeopathic reasoning! Ignorant of the agent causing smallpox, they proceeded by following the analogy between the morbid signs of the bovine vaccine and those of human smallpox (the responsible viruses of both are cousins), and had the idea of using the reactional defences mobilized by the first illness to create a protection from the second.

The next step was taken through Louis Pasteur's audacity in using the germ itself (the simile!), trying only to diminish its virulence. Of all modern vaccinations, only smallpox and tuberculosis remain similar in approach. The others have all become isopathic, in that the germ used is that of the human illness itself. Of course this is only a pale caricature of homoeopathy since without the dilution–potentization these elements are not elevated to the immaterial plane where the inspired Hahnemann had placed life itself. None the less, even without its energetic impact, the analogous reasoning is still a godsend since the great diseases that formerly terrorized our ancestors have now disappeared from the surface of the globe.

Unfortunately all good things can become noxious if their excessive use turns to abuse. Doctors should always measure the energetic impact of their interventions. Every vaccination is a shock, and any shock of this importance leaves a lasting immaterial mark on the impalpable space–time continuum, which animates the inert matter of our bodies. This trace can be extremely troublesome owing to the scarring effect imparted to the subtle cabling of our energetic transmissions, particularly when the physical body has not yet completed its growth. Misunderstanding this fact, the modern paediatrician behaves a bit like a bull in a china shop! The examples in the previous chapter are the unequivocal proof of these abuses.

Paediatricians vaccinate too soon, too abruptly, too closely together and against too many things at the same time. Dispensed too early, the vaccinal shock can create such a disharmony that a child will never recover the lost balance. You have only to imagine the complexity and the delicacy of the thousand secret ways in which vital energy seeps into all the structures of the tiny body as it develops, and you can understand to what extent such a brutal aggression can confuse the tenuous threads of health. As with my patients Benoît and the others mentioned earlier, the future becomes uncertain and frightening unless a real doctor can correct the resulting destinies. I regret that children are vaccinated before the age of 6 or 8 months since it is certain that their delicate systems of defence are not yet adequately developed to confront life in such a brutal manner. This is in fact the reason why their immunological protection is assured during the first months of life by the antibodies inherited from their mothers. But paediatrics scorns this maternal protection, which is judged insufficient and often incomplete (admittedly, often owing to the lack of breast feeding), and attempts to replace nature, administering its muzzled toxins in a now standardized schema that fixes D-Day at 3 months.

This premature assault is directly responsible for a second major calamity: the shock of surprise. How could a baby expect that the smiling, white-robed form will be the originator of the first serious disruption of its life? How could one alert the innocent vital energy? It will be taken by surprise, shaken to its roots, and can thus become destabilized.

These first two drawbacks of standard vaccinations are frequently enough in themselves to provoke the sinister imbalance. Unfortunately, the third flaw in the method only worsens things – the compulsory repetitions of the vaccinal intoxication, which are considered necessary to achieve adequate immunity. This is the well-known practice of 'booster shots' with its imperative and detailed calendar. I am not arguing against the findings of immunologists, which prove clearly the precarious nature of one-shot vaccinal protection. What I deplore is the fact that medicine uses only material vaccines to stimulate the antibodies. Each new shot introduces foreign bodies into the organism, the future consequences of which are unknown. Each booster is a new aggression that amplifies the first shock wave. And to these three disadvantages I will add a fourth concerning paediatrics – what has now become the classical mixture of three or four different toxins injected the same day at the same time. As I said earlier, nature would never permit such an aberration!

So how can one vaccinate without giving a shock to the system? Simple common sense dictates the answer. The method I use, outlined here, has always given complete satisfaction. First of all I no longer vaccinate before the 8th month because the mother's antibodies are more than sufficient to provide a first line of defence should illness occur, and fortunately breast feeding is once again fashionable. The only illness to be feared before that age is diphtheria. But here homoeopathy has an entire arsenal of powerful and very efficient remedies developed during the terrible years when diphtheria still raged. Allied with the natural immunity, these homoeopathic remedies are the best guardian angels of the first months of life.

How then do I vaccinate? The vaccination technique that I use is simple. Since vaccination is a shock, why not attenuate the shock by warning the defence systems a few days in advance? As I have already said, paediatricians vaccinate too abruptly, introducing more or less virulent toxins into a child's organism in a way not planned by nature and with no prior warning, in other words by breaking in. But this justified reproach disappears if I take the trouble to warn the guards by a false attack a few days before the real thing. To do this, I give the child a potency suited to the vaccinal nosode 2 or 3 days in advance (a dose at the 200th Korsakovian potency (*see* Glossary), or 200K is perfect). Thus the guards are alerted, the surprise effect is destroyed and on the day of the vaccination the enemy, already identified, is less of a problem. In practical terms, this leads to preservation of health, disharmony of energy is minimal and the antibodies develop more quickly.

And when should revaccination occur? My feeling is that 1 month after the initial intervention is the appropriate moment to ensure immunity. It is thus that I proceed by injecting the ordinary vaccine (this time without waving a warning flag with another dose at 200K because the immunity system has already been warned previously and therefore identifies the injected toxin with no problem). But I never recommend the third injection currently used by the majority of paediatricians. This third cumulative shock wave seems to me to be too dangerous at such a young age given the small gain in immunity that it achieves. I replace it advantageously by an enormous inverse shock, which I provoke by giving an oral dose of the vaccinal nosode taken to the fantastic strength of the 10,000K. Conscious of the strength of this shock I leave the child three days of 'active rest' before dealing this blow; (the 1st day the child receives a dose at 30K, the 2nd a dose at 200K and the 3rd day a much stronger dose at 1,000K. It is only on the fourth day that the high potency deploys its shock wave, modelling the immaterial support prepared by the three previous doses and which is already in a way vibrating in harmony with it.

The effects of this homoeopathic booster are wonderful. First of all, and most importantly, this immaterial booster erases for ever the terrible scar left on the vital energy by the vaccination. This return to harmony has an immediate effect on overall health as you can imagine from the examples I outlined in Chapter 10. Let me immediately reassure you (for people always ask me this question) that this homoeopathic erasure in no way removes the effect of the vaccination. In fact quite the contrary! And this is the second enormous advantage of the method: the immaterial shock is so powerful that our defence systems take it very seriously. These systems straight away set to work and produce large quantities of antibodies that confer a truly durable immunity on a child revaccinated in this manner. This immunity is very similar to that provoked by the illness itself, which rarely fails if it has struck strongly and completely. In this respect I think it is appropriate to assert that only children thus vaccinated are really vaccinated at all!

Naturally the transformation of this assertion into scientific doctrine would require periodic sampling of the antibodies. This has been done several times by certain homoeopaths and I have often verified the fact myself. It really does appear that an immunity created with a homoeopathic nosode lasts a lifetime. But a supplement to our documentation in the form of a major experimental study over a long period of time is still necessary. In 1980 I outlined a vast programme of study based on comparative analysis of a stable group of volunteers. I even managed to interest the Swiss military hierarchy, but it was impossible for me to bypass the 'scientific' commission comprised of well-known medical professionals entirely devoted to the powerful Swiss pharmaceutical lobby. However the file I prepared is still of interest and I would willingly put it at the disposal of any serious scientific group requesting it.

To summarize unequivocally the problem of vaccinations, I would say that children in the hands of modern paediatricians are overvaccinated, in other words excessively and badly, while those who go through the combination of vaccine and homoeopathy are well and truly 'pervaccinated'. I hope you will excuse the forging of these new words, but a word is often more expressive than a speech. I attach considerable importance to these explanations since in general the public imagines that homoeopaths are completely opposed to vaccinations. Perhaps some are, but for my part I am only opposed to the brutal and excessive manner in which modern medicine uses and abuses them. The practice of boosters decided upon blindly as a routine measure is also to be condemned. I believe that a more rigorous attitude is to determine before possible re-vaccination the proportion of antibodies in question. If they are in sufficient number, why then revaccinate? In saying this I realize that the methods employed to determine the correct number of antibodies are still costly and complex, but they are open to improvement and simplification.

Alas, only a handful of us base our work on these plain common-sense considerations. The doctrinaire fanaticism of the currently dominant materialist-based school is so strong that any opinion coming from another approach is summarily dismissed. Allopaths cannot tolerate the idea that an elite minority could one day teach in the faculties. They refuse to read our papers or allow them to be published in learned reviews. They are therefore unaware of the catastrophic effects of overvaccination on the system's energy equilibrium and instead are inclined to aggravate it.

In fact we are witnessing at the close of this 20th century a new phenomenon, unknown to preceding generations: childhood illnesses are becoming serious illnesses requiring extremely serious attention. I am not referring here to bacterial infections like scarlet fever or diphtheria, which doctors believe they have controlled with antibiotics, but to simple viral illnesses like mumps or measles. This may sound fantastic, but the fact is that common childhood measles could become a menace to the survival of our descendants. In all the countries of the civilized world there are cases (rare, one must admit) of encephalitis and other major complications following this illness. The paediatricians find it easy to terrorize mothers, then propose a vaccination, which is of course eagerly accepted.

What the doctors don't say (and don't even know) is that measles has become a serious illness through their own fault! They have so thoroughly managed to confuse the child's energy equilibrium that the innocent measles virus can get out of hand. Its attack on the body is easy because there is no resistance to overcome, and no defence. The same is true for the mumps virus, which can sometimes (very rarely) provoke serious glandular disturbance and even meningitis, or for any member of the large family of miscellaneous viruses that make a mockery of antibiotics.

But this is not the only problem with the current method of vaccinations. There is worse. By inoculating the baby with the measles toxin, paediatricians commit a major blunder. Have they ever really thought about what measles actually represents? In my opinion it is only anthroposophic medicine (*see* Glossary) in the West that has fully recognized the significance of childhood illnesses. According to Rudolf Steiner's followers, these are not really even 'illnesses', but rather the processes of maturing that nature has taken millennia to refine and which must respect a strict calendar. I think that they are right since this same thought process also exists in ancient Chinese medicine, so rich in important observations.

Let us go back to the example of measles. What do paediatricians do? They inoculate the virus before the age of 1 year. But nature has taken countless years to put together a process of measles to allow elimination through the skin of the excess energy remaining in the body following the first structural acquisitions of early childhood. It's a bit like a rocket, which drops its basic propulsion section once a certain height has been reached. Believe me, the natural process I describe above is as sophisticated and exactly timed as a NASA space project in all its details. The calendar of measles is precisely one of these details that cannot be neglected; the eruption must occur between infancy and childhood. Those tinkering with this wonderful safety valve are playing with fire. Who can say what enormous suffering this act of bravado may cause to humankind?

For the moment the official school triumphs. In 1982 the *Journal of the American Medical Association* jubilantly announced the enormous benefit to public health that vaccinations represented in terms of millions of dollars saved in medical expenses. It is true that short-term complications have declined significantly. But no one is thinking of the other complications: the treacherous distortions of vital energy. I'll be waiting for the enthusiastic author of the above article in twenty years to evaluate the damage ... unless of course the people who have been vaccinated read what follows and become adepts of 'real medicine'. In the mean time, yes, vaccinate the poor children in the developing countries of the world. Their vital energy is so weak that even a simple epidemic of measles could be fatal. Although it would logically be better just to feed them, the fact is that vaccination may save their lives. They are really the only beneficiaries of this new technique. All the other children that I have dealt with have suffered at its hands.

As an illustration, let me tell the story of David F, born in 1981, a typical example of dozens of other cases I have treated concerning this particularly sinister form of overvaccination. When I first saw him on 6 February 1984 he had been running a fever for 7 weeks. It appeared to have been caused by otitis, which was diagnosed by the paediatrician, but continued despite treatment with antibiotics! The ever-present Clamoxyl had been abandoned after 7 days owing to an obvious allergic reaction. Various anti-inflammatory drugs (since fever is a sign of inflammation) had since been tried with no greater effect(!). The treatment seemed very straightforward since the child had been troubled in his short life only by the ear problem and the iatrogenic intoxication from vaccinations and chemical medication. So I started the therapeutic sequence by cleaning out the antibiotic traces from the hepatic–biliary system. The next step was to administer on 20 February the nosodes of the only vaccination that the child's records indicated: DTPP. Sure of myself, I predicted the anticipated drop in temperature ... and was totally wrong. The miserable little fever continued to defy me and all my wonderful homoeopathic remedies throughout March and April. Before jumping to conclusions I asked the mother whether the child had been vaccinated against measles. Her answer was in the negative, and I began to despair. The child's temperature was already at 39.5°C (103°F). Luckily the truth came out in May when the mother finally discovered that the measles vaccination had indeed occurred.

On 18 May, with the fever at 39°C (102°F), I administered Morbillinum, the missing nosode in the sequential puzzle. What followed was so simple that the story ends here. Health, like an electric light, returned the moment the switch was turned back on.

Every bit as modern is the mumps vaccination. It is generally associated with the vaccination just discussed in the same unnatural spirit of rapid simplification. German measles is often also given at the same time as a triple combined vaccination which has managed to enchant our more up-to-date colleagues. Although not as dangerous as the measles inoculation, this parotitic overvaccination can create an enormous and sometimes irreparable energetic disturbance, particularly in 'phosphoric' constitutions. This concept is entirely specific to homoeopathy and unfortunately remains completely unknown to allopaths. This is a shame since knowledge of the different constituent elements of our personalities is very enriching to the art of healing.

Our teacher often compared the homoeopathic doctor to a good gardener who is able to recognize the different types of fruit trees in his garden and knows the right treatment for each one. In contrast the allopathic doctor only sees trees and applies the same treatment to all of them. This is really the best way to describe the current mania for vaccinations, which give the same doses of the same vaccines at the same dates to all children with no reference at all to the diversity of their constitutions.

But let's go back to our phosphoric type. In homoeopathic teaching, this is the definition given to a slender person, often thin and active, perhaps even agitated, often bohemian or artistic but none the less respectful of established authority, etc. Phosphorics are quite sensitive to any attacks on the integrity of their endocrine systems. Well, mumps invade the parotid glands, the pancreas and the sexual glands with a retroactive effect on all other centres of hormonal regulation. This inoculation can have incalculable consequences on this type of person, causing for example the appearance several months later of a sudden and inexplicable obesity or significant loss of weight or even a marked depression, diabetes, perturbed growth or menstrual cycles, loss of hair, and so on.

This is a pretty high price to pay for a very relative protection against a virus that is not as bad as its reputation leads us to believe, particularly when a doctor can take care of it in our way.

As for whooping cough, I do not understand why there are still paediatricians around who recommend inoculating against it. First of all, the illness is not very dangerous and can even be useful in exercising the immune system. In addition, it has been proved a thousand times that the vaccine is not very efficient since there are countless numbers of vaccinated children who fall ill anyway. Lastly, a small but often noted detail, children who are ill despite the vaccination cough endlessly day and night. I've noticed this so often that I formally and systematically advise all parents who ask me to avoid this additional and useless overvaccination.

Unfortunately, mothers are often deceived by their paediatricians. They may ask in a pleasant way that this vaccination not be given, but practitioners are either so stuck in their routine or their stocks are so large that such requests are sometimes completely ignored.

The story of Nicholas J is a case in point. This child was brought to my office on 20 December 1983 for the reason you may have guessed: he coughed and coughed endlessly and had done so for weeks. Examination by his allopathic doctor had found no visible reason for the bothersome and worrying problem. The mother, who had requested to the paediatrician that her son not be inoculated with this useless toxin, had asked me for the nosodes required to remove vaccinal traces following the second DiTePol vaccination. No other event had yet occurred to trouble the stream of the child's life. But with the ohmmeter I found an obvious blockage of the Lung meridian and the child's vaccination records quickly showed me the source of the problem: the paediatrician had injected four times DiTePerPol (Per for Pertussis – whooping cough) instead of the DiTePol requested. The logical treatment (several progressively increased potencies of the appropriate nosode) quickly replaced the numerous cough syrups and restored Nicholas's health.

There is another classical variation to this banal observation, which the story of Julien L born in 1977 will illustrate. The facts are as follows. The child had coughed since infancy and no treatment had been able to cure the chronic bronchitis diagnosed by the paediatrician. At 4 months, his parents took him to the south of the Alps for 4 weeks in the hope that a change of climate would improve things. Unfortunately the air in the Ticino was no better than that of the Jura and no progress occurred. Back at home the coughing continued and the doctor's 'anti' drugs along with it. Several cases of otitis, the removal of his adenoids and finally of his tonsils (something had to be done after all!) all failed to solve the problem and the bronchitis appeared to be firmly anchored. In October 1983 the paediatrician decided to have blood tests done which are both costly and essentially worthless, because the doctor doesn't know how to use them to their full extent. If he had only been able to step beyond archaic allopathic reasoning he would have found the solution as quickly as I did. The analyses clearly showed the way. Along with the ordinary viruses was the guilty party: the whooping cough bacillus. The mother provided the complete list of disruptive events: BCG at 1 month, DTPP four times between 3 and 8 months, measles overvaccination at 16 months, mumps at the age of 2 years, followed by German measles and finally a real case of whooping cough at age 6 despite the three booster shots received!

On the ohmmeter all the meridians were correctly balanced except the Lung, which was seriously affected. I started my liberating treatment with the most recent event, the whooping cough, but cautiously gave only a medium potency of the Pertussinum nosode since I was not trying to erase the four whooping cough shocks of the first months. The child's cough worsened with this first attack, but I didn't give way to impatience and proceeded in the proper sequence: Varicellinum, Parotidinum, Morbillinum, and finally the real guilty parties, the four DTPPs and the sinister BCG (which was in fact the major destabilizer of the entire story). The child had almost entirely stopped coughing since taking Morbillinum, but as soon as he took the DTPP nosode (this time at a high potency) a terrible cough began and lasted 3 days. It was like the finale of a fireworks display and he has never coughed since. Why should he? His restored vital energy has regained control of the Lung meridian and he is now completely cured.

To close this chapter on childhood overvaccination, I must say a word about German measles. At first glance the idea of vaccinating against such a harmless and widespread illness seems grotesque to any doctor with an ounce of common sense. Indeed, the idea is ridiculous, particularly if the vaccination is administered during the first months of life in some 'modern' and unnatural combined multiple inoculation. But it is important to remember what terrible fetal deformations this virus can provoke during the first 3 months of a pregnancy. The widespread vaccination of girls therefore seems highly justified, with one reservation, that a check is done first to see whether the illness has perhaps already occurred in childhood.

Diagnosis of German measles is fairly simple since it is the only short eruptive illness (the rash only lasts 3 days) with very characteristic ganglionary signs behind the ears, at the back of the neck and sometimes even higher up near the scalp. It is nevertheless often not diagnosed because the doctor either is not consulted or hesitates to define the illness. This is why the safest and wisest approach in the absence of a clear memory of the illness, and particularly if no antibodies are found, is to vaccinate young girls. Three days before inoculation I give Rubeolinum 200K and again 3 weeks later, this time going all the way up to 10,000K. This is the best guarantee against an eventual reawakening of this capricious and dangerous virus.

As you can see, this isopathic concept of immunization is at considerable variance with the misleading doctrine presented by the official schools of medicine. For them it is theoretically possible to protect against all infectious illness. All you have to do is isolate the responsible agent and diminish its virulence before injecting it. Since the procedure isn't natural, the resulting immunity is not perfect and doesn't last. That's why periodic revaccination is required.

You can now see the serious flaws in this method. On the one hand it is not very reliable, and on the other it is very aggressive. The overvaccination destabilizes the baby's vital energy, opening the door to the various morbid possibilities of adult life that we have so modestly baptized 'illnesses of civilization'.

Instead of receding, these illnesses will become more and more diversified and will appear in forms that are presently unknown to our clinicians unless this 'progress' is urgently halted. In the United States there is already discussion about vaccinating children against chicken-pox and scarlet fever, while certain people are even quite calmly proposing that children be vaccinated while still in their mother's womb! Is a public health disaster going to be necessary to bring medicine back to its senses or will common sense triumph? It is not really all that difficult to comply with nature's requirements. She knows the correct steps to take in all circumstances and asks only for a little support, particularly during the first years of life. All one has to do is let these childhood illnesses 'come out', directing only the reactional modalities of the young patient with the help of homoeopathy. I will explain how to do this later. And for more serious illnesses such as polio, smallpox or tetanus, the only real immunization comes through the energetic activation of the vaccine using a correctly potentized homoeopathic nosode.

This supporting of the material vaccine by its immaterial nosode is the essence, indeed the definition, of 'pervaccination', a technique at the forefront of 'Real Medicine'.

TWELVE

Genetic pollution

We have just seen the enormous responsibility of modern paediatrics in destabilizing children's vital energy for a problematic improvement in protection which in every sense of the term is paid at too high a price. The devastating effects of overvaccination have not yet been recognized by official medicine. Homoeopaths haven't made an inventory of them all either. In fact, only the tiny minority of colleagues familiar with the ohmmetric technique or the Chinese pulses have fully recognized the binary nature of vital energy. Even rarer are doctors capable of appreciating the nature of the disturbances.

In the examples cited earlier, all the allopaths have failed miserably because they missed the only important diagnosis: that of energetic imbalance. Most of the classic Hahnemannian or Kentian homoeopaths would have also failed because it is pointless to hope for a reactional adaptation until the mutilated vital energy has been freed by the correct therapeutic sequence.

But what I showed you in these first examples was only a first glimpse, lacking a detailed analysis of the real significance of the different vaccinal shocks. I must now be more specific. First of all, it is possible to make the essential distinction between vaccinations that protect against childhood illnesses and vaccinations that make superior claims. In the first group, I put diphtheria, whooping cough, measles, German measles and mumps; in the second, BCG (a tuberculosis vaccination), tetanus, polio, smallpox, rabies, cholera, typhus, and yellow fever. In one group you can recognize the common 'childhood' illnesses; in the other are the much more serious diseases, which are also fortunately much rarer.

I would have liked to present you with a group of patients that had come to a breaking point in their energetic balance merely as a result of the first vaccinations, but unfortunately it is impossible nowadays to find a child who has not had one or more vaccinations from the second group as well. As a result, nobody can predict the amplitude of imbalance created solely by these 'infant' vaccinations. Reasoning can, however, make up for the lack of documentation. It is possible to imagine that without the TePol element, the hammering from the DiPer vaccine would have been adequate to make little Nicholas cough all his life; Julien would perhaps have had the same thing occurring without the TePol and BCG toxins. You could also speculate in like manner about any of the other young patients that I have presented. I chose these stories precisely because these anamneses were not overly encumbered with vaccinations from the second group.

Through this first selection, you have a glimpse of the destabilization that is fairly representative of an ideal model that cannot be found. If we now analyse these first examples, certain things become evident: the imbalance that has been introduced is not what one would call inhuman since the incriminating shocks are only ersatz versions for what in essence are quite ordinary events. Diphtheria, whooping cough, measles, mumps, German measles are not, in themselves, an affront to our human condition. We must all pass through these stages of maturation; this has been so for thousands of years ... By artificially introducing morbid information into the guiding systems of an infant, the paediatrician is only advancing the inevitable moment of natural recognition. Childhood epidemics have existed throughout history. They occur every year, taking their allotted toll of victims. Rare are the children who escape this phenomenon. Humanity suffers the hammer blows of these periodic explosions, which systematically leave their imprints on our genetic code.

By vaccinating in an untimely manner (too early, too abruptly, too often and too many at a time), the paediatrician is merely awakening in a severe way an underlying and common imprint. The protective gesture would seem almost to be harmless since everything is taking place in known terrain, between germs and viruses on good terms with each other, so to speak. One would suppose that the vital energy shouldn't take umbrage.

Unfortunately, as we have just seen, this is not the case. It is more susceptible than one might think, and no one knows the calamities that can be caused by this initial well-intentioned error.

What then can be said about the second type of vaccinal intoxication? Tetanus, cholera, poliomyelitis, smallpox, etc are not ordinary illnesses that everyone is supposed to have had as a matter of course. Clearly the serious infectious diseases have burdened humanity from time immemorial, but their periodic explosions are fortunately not as frequent as are childhood illnesses. The marks that remain imprinted on our genetic memories are less pronounced and are perhaps even partly erased in the case of certain widespread epidemics which even the doctors have forgotten. Logically it would seem safe to assume that the vaccinal shock will be more violent for such illnesses given the fact that our organisms no longer recognize these enemies from a past age. We find here the surprise effect mentioned above, which we have seen to be capable of significantly affecting the delicate balance of vital energy.

But this is not the only reason to be prudent in using these toxins. There is a double danger in vaccinating against these terrible and rare diseases since the medical act is in this case purely artificial. On the one hand, it renders commonplace, by generalization and repetition, a situation that nature in no way wanted to make widespread. Who can know the consequences of this bravado? Can doctors be certain that the repeated injection of the tetanus toxin does not modify, over a period of time, from parents to children, our genetic structure itself? On the other hand, the act in my opinion comes close to sheer thoughtlessness when a doctor inoculates a human child with toxins that are animal in nature. The fact is that, for most vaccines, the toxin is that of the illness itself. In vaccinating against childhood illnesses, doctors are merely introducing information that belongs to mankind. For greater protection they limit themselves to the inoculation of a diminished germ of the illnesses that our species can contract. But in intervening against certain other dangerous illnesses, doctors cannot use human toxins; they then inoculate animal toxins by analogy. The iatrogenic pollution is therefore more violent since it is not at all certain that these animal fragments belong to the ancient inheritance of our ultimate genetic constituents. Introducing them without precaution into our ancestral baggage, in other words without the superior control of homoeopathy, risks profoundly modifying our most innermost structures. In the prevention of serious infectious diseases the risk of dangerously altering the delicate immaterial wiring of our energetic transmissions is therefore doubled. To help you understand better the extent of this menace I will now present the star of these diseases: the dreaded smallpox.

SMALLPOX

Without going into the entire history of this scourge, I must remind you that before the introduction of systematic prevention, which was fully completed at the end of the last century, smallpox killed several tens of thousands of people in Europe every year. Since then this prophylaxis has been extended over the entire planet to such an extent that the World Health Organization has recently spoken of its complete eradication and has ceased recommending obligatory vaccination. With the exception of very young children we have therefore all, including parents, grandparents and possibly even their parents, been vaccinated against smallpox. Do you believe this triple or quadruple impregnation has been totally innocent? I'm not so sure, because any energetic intervention (the vaccine is a shock!) leaves its mark on the superior space–time continuum which animates the lineage of our successive physical bodies. Yes, one must recognize once and for all that vital energy is unlimited and infinite like the entity that gives birth to it. It doesn't stop with our death, and a part of its informational vibrations insinuates itself in the genetic patrimony of our descendants with each generation. Ancient China had clearly identified this element of our vital energy, so aptly baptized 'ancestral energy'.

You find it hard to believe that a vaccination is capable of modifying our genetic baggage? You think that such a common act is incapable of such long-term consequences? While not calling the biologists in as witnesses, who advance scientific proof expressing the same opinion, I will enlighten you without embarking upon a boring course of molecular biophysics. I will merely present hard, undisputed facts and let them speak for themselves.

The following story should convince you that the small scarification inflicted on your plump infantile arm has marked you for life. I know the story very well since it is mine. It is very instructive, and it is important that I recount it. Like all children born in French Indochina, I received the primary smallpox vaccination in the first few weeks of my life. This initial scarification didn't result in the usual blister, which indicates that the vaccination has 'taken'. I was therefore revaccinated. The colonial health authorities were not to be taken lightly! But once again the vaccination didn't take. I don't know how many times my parents had to present me to the doctors in question, but they finally desisted given that my skin remained intact despite their best efforts. Not the slightest scar appeared! I managed to escape all attempts at revaccination for 40 years.

One day in Lausanne I received a notice from the local health officials recommending that all doctors be revaccinated because an epidemic had broken out 400 kilometres from our borders, in the Balkans. Obedient, I went upstairs to a neighbouring colleague and asked him to revaccinate me against smallpox. Finding no trace on my skin of the first vaccinations he hesitated, rightly considering that I had no immunity. In this case, the vaccination would be a primary vaccination, and everyone knows that such an enterprise is hazardous for an adult since it can cause dangerous complications. I none the less reassured him about my history of vaccinations, and he re-did the well-known scarification in the usual place on the upper part of the left arm in the middle of the deltoid muscle.

I waited 3, 4, then 8 days. Nothing happened. Once again, the vaccine hadn't taken!

Shortly thereafter, I met Dr Senn, began my homoeopathic apprenticeship and somewhat later experimented on myself with the sequential method that I had discovered. When I reached smallpox, I was prepared for anything since I had proof of the vaccine and its complete inefficacity. I took the smallpox nosode ... and it didn't take long for things to start happening. Beginning with the MK (1,000th Korsakovian) potency, and even worse after the XMK, (10,000th potency) I had one of the worst attacks of lumbosciatica that I have ever encountered. I was completely paralysed. My wife had to drive me to the office and I could only with difficulty get out of the car. I couldn't walk alone. This pleasant interlude lasted 1 day before giving way to the terrible diarrhoea that took its place.

I was going to forget the entire episode when 6 or 7 days later I felt the curious need to scratch my left shoulder at the top of my arm. I looked in the mirror at the place of the itch and to my stupefaction discovered the incredible phenomenon: before my eyes was appearing the classical smallpox blister of a primary vaccination! And it evolved over the next few days exactly like all vaccinal blisters, gradually reaching a slightly watery purulence, drying and finally leaving a very clear and perfectly indelible little scar.

But the final message of this story is that the vaccination (finally!) 'took' at exactly the same spot as the very first vaccination which I had received as a small child, and not at the place of the most recent scarification. Proof of this is the characteristic location at the very top of the arm, almost on the shoulder. It is certainly not there that my colonial paediatrician had vaccinated me for the first time. Just like my more recent colleague, he had used the appropriate place on the protrusion of the deltoid muscle. But everyone knows that the topography of a child's scars changes with growth. Just like the bark of a tree, the skin doesn't necessarily follow the more rapid growth of the underlying structure. Scars, like the intertwined hearts on the surface of the wood, can often be found in a location different from that where they first took place.

This observation is interesting in more than one respect. First of all, it proves irrefutably that a correctly potentized homoeopathic nosode has the fantastic ability to go back in time and reawaken a past energetic event all the way to the site of its original physical manifestation. That is not bad for a placebo! Secondly, it shows that only the primary vaccination seems to be important since the awakening of the dormant biological process didn't arouse the later toxic deposits. I have had confirmation of this phenomenon several times since, and it is always a delicate moment in the sequential therapy to know how to pinpoint exactly in time the first marking event in an analogous sequence. (I earlier gave you an example with little Julien's whooping cough.)

Finally, this adventure should make even the doubting Thomases understand that any vaccination is a major act irremedially modifying our ways of reacting, even if the direct consequences are insignificant or even invisible.

As striking as this example of materialization through the immaterial may be, it still only provides first-degree proof of the 'ethereal' permanence of any event, because the activity of the energetic distortion lasts here only the ridiculous space of a short lifetime. Yet it seems that an important event can leave a much more marked trail that is capable of disturbing the energetic regulation of successive generations. Once again, it is smallpox that will provide a dramatic demonstration of this assertion.

At the beginning of my career as a homoeopath, I corrected the energetic distortions following smallpox vaccination in the manner taught by Dr Senn, using the nosode Variolinum. All of his students do the same. However, on reflection, Variolinum is the nosode of smallpox itself, the terrifying disease so feared by all doctors. Their fear of this scourge is so great that they have never dared to vaccinate using a strain of the virus itself. That is why a less-virulent strain is used: that of cowpox. Vaccinating doctors are actually imitating homoeopathy without realizing it as they are injecting a 'similar' virus.

Both Senn and his students, by giving Variolinum to those vaccinated with the vaccine, are also giving the most 'similar' nosode. But it is obvious that it is possible to do even better: by giving the nosode of the vaccine itself, called Vaccinotoxinum, its perfect isotherapeutic. As we have already seen, the correction of an imbalance is incomparably more efficient if the nosode used is that of the causal agent itself.

It was only after grasping this truth that I was able to understand what had happened to little Paloma S, whom I saw during the first months of my homoeopathic practice in 1975. The short anamnesis of this 4-year-old child only mentioned the usual vaccinations and the smallpox vaccine. The cleaning up of her toxic past was quickly done and I had just completed the final touches with the Variolinum nosode corresponding to the first shock of her life. Several days later the mother called in a panic: her daughter's body was covered with horrible oozing blisters! I saw the child immediately and the mother was right, the sight was frightening: face and body covered with the characteristic smallpox sores. In giving the Variolinum nosode I had unwittingly reawakened a toxic permeation that was much older than the vaccine, which after all was only inoculated cowpox. And then I found the key to the mystery. The child's grandmother had almost succumbed to a terrible smallpox epidemic from which she retained the disfiguring scars all her life. To avoid a similar destiny, her daughter had been vaccinated at birth (with a strong feverish reaction) and the granddaughter had been put through the same ritual despite the end of obligatory vaccination against smallpox.

By giving Variolinum as my teacher had taught me, I had clumsily jumped straight over the child and mother's vaccinations and right into the middle of the smallpox target, the real smallpox of the grandmother. Luckily the healing homoeopathic shock is more spectacular than damaging, and little Paloma's smooth childhood skin returned a few days later. But this adventure had opened my eyes to a terrible reality: an important event can imprint its mark with a red-hot iron, like a biblical curse, on an entire lineage. I will never forget that lovely child's face momentarily disfigured with pockmarks, and you can well understand the fear I now have of biological 'brandings' invented by Dame Medicine.

No one can convince me that repeated lifelong impregnations of rare and barbarous toxins do not alter the complex play of genetic transmission. We are in fact already paying for these apprentice-sorcerer's experiments with a very real impoverishment of the human race. I will come back to this point later. For the moment I must draw your attention to a third fact: vaccinal manipulations not only modify our etheric bodies and those of our descendants, but also the visible structures of our physical bodies.

In proof of this here is another sad example from the smallpox files. Everyone knows of the dreadful cellulitis of the buttocks and thighs that can grotesquely deform the silhouette of certain unfortunate young women. Mother Nature, the inventor of graceful feminine curves, certainly did not intend this cruel disfiguration. Like all monstrosities, this caricature was imposed on her by some form of violence. Here once again the problem is the result of the doctors and their good intentions.

When Dr Senn informed us that this unhappy condition can be the direct consequence of a smallpox vaccination we didn't want to believe him at first. However I was shortly afterwards able to verify his surprising assertion. Denise M, a young woman from Lausanne, came to see me in December 1975 suffering from a bad case of flu. I had treated her 2 years earlier for a distressing tendency towards repetitive cases of thrombophlebitis, which I had been able to stop using serocytol therapy. This time she was again afraid for her legs which were already rather sore from the recent stay in bed. The unfortunate young woman had already intrigued me on account of the solid mass of cellulitis from the waist down that disfigured an otherwise slender and attractive figure. At the time I didn't know the reason, not having been taught it by the faculty, and all my attempts at a cure had failed despite the insistence of my patient.

But I now had a new weapon, the smallpox nosode, and if our teacher was right this deformation should quickly disappear following its prescription. Unhesitatingly, and in total contradiction to the sequential logic that I had yet to discover, I gave her the famous 'placebo' potentized to a very high strength. It was only 5 months later that I again saw my patient, for a small problem of a totally different nature. Radiant, she showed me her now perfectly normal thighs! The only treatment had been the smallpox nosode, and the cellulitis had melted away as if by magic. Here again is proof that an apparently harmless vaccine can also modify the visible structures of our physical bodies for life.

There remains one last subject of concern, which is treated as lightly as the others by the men in white. I refer here to the place on the body where the vaccination is administered, the importance of which no study I have seen has ever spoken. Let us go back to our smallpox example and you will quickly understand the reasons for my perplexity.

For people of a certain age, the location of the smallpox vaccination is easily found owing to the enormous marks left on the upper arm on either side of the median line in a double scar, oval and very ugly. Why this double trace? Because at the time it was common to vaccinate by double scarification since the stability of the product was not always guaranteed. But, by proceeding in this manner, the doctor inadvertently spared the Chinese meridian which is critical to the Large Intestine, and which passes precisely on the outside of the arm along the median line. Unfortunately, people of my generation were no longer so lucky. Since the 1930s, the vaccinal strains used are considerably more stable, and doctors no longer perform the vaccination in two parts. One scarification is enough, and now it is right in the middle of the arm directly on top of the Chinese meridian corresponding to the Large Intestine.

I have often wondered if the extraordinary increase in intestinal and colonic cancers observed over recent decades is not somehow related to this vaccination practice. Naturally it would not be the main cause, but is perhaps an important triggering mechanism, particularly given that men are more affected than women. With women, the current aesthetic criteria have progressively convinced doctors to mark the skin in less visible places than the upper arm. They presently use the upper thigh, which is crossed only by the Gall Bladder meridian which fortunately curves slightly at that place and is thus more protected from this medical act.

These and other considerations have led me to believe that the location of a vaccination can play a hidden but very important role in the formation of a number of clinical tendencies, a role entirely ignored by our Western medicine. This increasing impression became a certitude the day that chance brought me a case that was so evident that my last doubts vanished. Here is the strange story.

In June 1981 a young woman aged 30 came to my office. She was a dancer and was suffering from persistent and intense migraine headaches. As she listed her miseries I was immediately struck by the incredible repetitions of renal colic, which had been ruining her life for years. It isn't surprising when a patient who is predisposed to having kidney stones has an occasional crisis. That is fairly common. But surely if the crises continue endlessly, any doctor should try to go beyond sympathizing and bringing relief. An attempt at stretching his knowledge becomes imperative.

So I systematically explored the Kidney meridian and to my amazement found an enormous scar from smallpox vaccination (again!) on the inside of the ankle which was completely suffocating the third and fourth points of the meridian. The acupuncturists I questioned were unable to provide an explanation of the eventual cause-and-effect relationship, but simple common sense obliged me to refute the notion that this was mere chance. I started my retroactive sequential treatment, and it took a year for me to reach the time-frame of the primary smallpox vaccination. I administered a high potency of the vaccinal nosode on 9 August 1982 ... and the patient was delivered from her nightmare. She ceased producing the little crystals of calcium oxalates that had caused her so much pain.

From that day on I was totally convinced. Any vaccination profoundly changes our energetic balance, our genetic code and our morphology itself, as much through the nature of the shock itself as through the moment and the place where it is administered. It is essential that this be known to all doctors and never forgotten.

I don't want to be tiresome, dear reader, but I deem it necessary to list some other unpleasant occurrences (great and small) that can be caused to some unfortunate people by vaccinations of the second category. How did I establish this list? Simply by observing the different consecutive reactions of elimination and adaptation when taking the corresponding nosodes.

To finish with the smallpox vaccination, here is a summary of its effects.

- It always disturbs the hydromineral balance of the tissues and can be considered one of the most active hidden factors causing cellulitis, from an unwanted change of shape to a terrible disfiguration.
- It is the hidden cause of innumerable cases of lumbago and sciatica that return throughout the year despite the best manual care and without the slightest sign of mechanical lesion.
- It can be one of the subtle causes of intestinal cancer and of the frequent and modern feminine pathology of the gall bladder.
- It was the responsible agent in the fairly numerous cases of incurable sterility which I have had the joy of curing.
- It provokes countless skin and mucous diseases that are worsened in summer, as well as the classic meningeal

symptoms that are well known in ordinary medicine. Certain chronic headaches sometimes have no other cause.
- It can definitively alter one or another quality of the blood and can play a determinant role in what is referred to as 'essential' hypertension owing to ignorance of its causes.

This litany is only a brief overview of the main perverse aptitudes of this demonic vaccine. For each of these statements, I could give you examples from my daily practice. But a tiresome list of the miseries of others would resemble too closely those first stories that you had the patience to read in Chapters 10 and 11. My treatment plan never changes and its continued reiteration would be superfluous.

I always proceed in the same manner, first determining the chronological order of the key events that I feel have played a 'marking' role in the space–time continuum of my patient, then going back in time with the appropriate sequence of the most similar nosodes. Once I reach the primary vaccination episode, I give the corresponding nosode and observe a regression of the observed pathological signs, frequently preceded by a momentary worsening of the symptoms.

In the smallpox example, the cellulitis increases then regresses, the digestive problems worsen then disappear, the menstrual cycle is troubled then returns to normal, eczema, herpes or impetigo blossom then wither, etc. By minute observation of these reactions, 'isosequential' homoeopathy contributes to inventorying specific morbid troubles and permits the establishment of very interesting relationships of cause and effect.

For each marking event, the homoeopath creates a catalogue of visible consequences observed during the energetic correction of the nosode. This simple technique is a wonderful source of invaluable information. It is unfortunately totally unknown to the vast majority of the medical profession, to the great detriment of all patients.

TETANUS

I think I have covered the most important aspects of this first vaccination, so useful and pernicious, and whose invention goes back to the beginning of time. But what of the second more modern one, which claims to protect us from tetanus, that other terrible scourge that generally kills its victims?

It is probably as useful as the first, since we can point to far fewer deaths since the entire population of our civilized countries has been vaccinated. Unfortunately this protection is also purchased at a high price since the reiterated introduction of tetanus toxin into our organisms provokes a very clear energetic imbalance that allopaths can neither see nor correct. Homoeopaths themselves frequently ignore the effects, since the clinical signs of this iatrogenic pollution are so ordinary that only those who are familiar with isotherapy know how to find them. Here are two of those effects, which my teacher indicated to all his students and that I have observed countless times myself.

The first, found in almost all tetanus overvaccinations, affects the neuromuscular system. Victims suffer from various cramps, increased fatigue following exercise, inhabitual stiffness of the support structure of the cervical column. The chewing muscles are clenched, the physiognomy is tense. Classical night-time cramps, like most other manifestations of tetany, often have no other cause. One hears a lot nowadays about tetany and books are written about this fashionable illness. You can skip reading them if you correct your tetanic overvaccination with the adequate nosode!

The second, unexpected, will surprise you: it is baldness – not the baldness of old people or that of the unfortunate persons carrying a gene causing premature baldness, but rather the one involving the slow and inexorable process afflicting so many unfortunate young men early in life. As if by chance, this misfortune frequently starts with the beginning of military service and I have often heard helmets blamed as the originating cause of the problem. Some manage to console themselves by attributing this disfavour to their exceptional virility ... But reality is far more prosaic. Induction into the army generally implies a massive intoxication with the tetanus toxin, which has become compulsory in all the world's armies. The lucky ones, protected by their genetic constellation or by homoeopathy, escape this humiliation; the others resign themselves to it.

They should none the less be reassured. If they entrust the regulation of their energetic balance to a doctor familiar with isotherapy, they will be able to avoid complete baldness if they still have enough hair follicles left at the beginning of the treatment. Here also they will lose hair by the fistful after receiving the tetanus nosode – this is the classic homoeopathic aggravation – but their mood will improve once they recognize that the phenomenon has stopped and the hair is growing back.

The vaccine has other disagreeable surprises in store, concerning the electrolytic balance, kidney functions and endocrine harmony. It is not my goal to list all these problems here since this book is not intended to be a medical treatise. But the reader should know that vaccinal protection is always purchased at a high price if it is not followed by a rigorous isopathic cleansing.

POLIOMYELITIS

After smallpox and tetanus, poliomyelitis is the disease that most terrorizes civilized populations and their doctors. Clearly it doesn't kill as assuredly as the other two, but the evocation of its crippling and almost incurable after-effects strikes fear into people's hearts and minds. When Dr Salk invented his vaccine it was therefore an immense relief to the entire medical profession, who were thrilled at this new victory over fatality. Sadly, the triumph was short lived. It became very quickly evident that the technique was flawed, and thousands of victims sacrificed their health to excessive haste in seeking protection. The public was not on the whole informed, nor indeed were the doctors, but this dangerous intramuscular vaccination was surreptitiously replaced with the Sabin oral vaccine, which was declared viable and perfectly safe.

In my radiesthesic readings I often come upon the energetic imbalance caused by the Salk vaccine. I erase the morbid spatiotemporal trace with the poliomyelitis nosode and this correction usually causes headaches, muscular pain, diarrhoea and sometimes fever. Such a flare-up of symptoms is the unquestionable proof of the extremely toxic nature of the intramuscular vaccination.

This retrospective proof is damning because it signifies that millions of human beings are still carrying this deadly toxin and the etheric stigma of its imprint. No one thinks about releasing them from it. The vaccine was discreetly 'withdrawn from the market', and victims' families were quietly indemnified, but the immense majority of those vaccinated will forever carry the dangerous traces of it ... unless the medical profession emerges from its academic torpor and finally rediscovers medicine.

Here again, the younger generations have been fortunate. Since 1958, the oral Sabin vaccination has replaced its rival. It is undoubtedly less dangerous and has solicited only minor opposition, even among homoeopaths. Nevertheless, certain children still have an intolerance to it, and I now recommend that all my patients tell me of any muscular pain, headaches or vague digestive trouble occurring shortly after a Sabin vaccination. If such is the case, I give them the poliomyelitis nosode also, and am sometimes surprised to awaken the same symptoms as those occurring in people freed from the Salk.

It also happens that adults are bothered by the Sabin. This summer I saw Sylviane P from Yverdon, a young woman aged 19, who had received her first oral vaccination in March 1984. During the following days her neck became swollen, the glands became enormous and painful, the tonsils started playing up, and the nape of the neck was sore. She suffered from extreme muscular pain in the legs and lower back, and was overcome by intense exhaustion lasting over a month. Despite this warning, her doctor had the impudence to give her another oral dose the following month – which naturally created the same troubling series of reactions.

I saw her at the end of July. The body's key meridian was clearly affected by this iatrogenic shock, and my first action (you've probably guessed) was to erase this last insult to her energetic balance with the poliomyelitis nosode.

As you can see from this example, a healthy caution is the best guide in the administration of this third important vaccine. As with smallpox or tetanus, the polio vaccination should not be imposed on our defence systems without prior warning to them. I remain convinced that the faculty will one day have to accept the homoeopaths' convincing arguments and abandon overvaccinating in favour of the more logical rules of pervaccinating with nosodes.

TROPICAL INFECTIONS

With these three major vaccinations of the second group, intended to protect us from illnesses unplanned in our genetic baggage, the major part of vaccination dangers has been covered. But the fashion for travel to exotic countries has created a new source of medical concern and in so doing a new form of iatrogenic pollution. I refer here to the tropical vaccinations that many of our contemporaries have before visiting countries where typhus, typhoid fevers, cholera and yellow fever are rampant. These unusual toxins constitute an enormous danger for our energetic equilibrium and should at all cost be counterbalanced by the corresponding isopathic nosodes. I have myself experienced the degree to which the vaccinal shock of cholera can compromise the physical harmony of a life from childhood to maturity, and I cannot recommend too highly to all travellers that they have these exotic toxins conscientiously removed when they return home.

Clearly life and even health are possible without such a perfectionist rectification. But one feels so much better after this homoeopathic cleansing! Why deprive oneself of this easy cure when knowing that the energetic effect of vaccinal intoxication can last an entire lifetime? Why run the risk of ageing badly when knowing that chronic illness is merely the signature of a chronic imbalance? In speaking of deregulation (not of airlines!), I can assure you that tropical vaccinations take first prize! It would be hard to imagine greater troublemakers. I have already encountered a variety of the miseries they produce – a slender child who becomes obese after three cholera injections, another who becomes diabetic or paralysed, a businessman who can't recover from a trip prepared for by his doctor, a young explorer who wastes away following preventative measures against yellow fever. I could give you so many examples but you would only really believe me the day you had the experience yourselves.

Before closing this pessimistic chapter, I still must share one last thought inspired by association with germs and exotic viruses. In Lausanne I rarely have occasion to take care of people from faraway countries. That is why I am particularly attentive when the occasion arises.

This is the story of Jean-Claude A, a 3-year-old black boy from Dahomey whose adoptive family brought him to me in the summer of 1976 because he had become very unruly since his last tropical vaccination. The truth is that he was frankly unbearable! He wouldn't sit still, and was climbing all over the furniture, looking at me in a surly way and disrupting the world around him with frightening, inexplicable and violent fits of anger.

I started the sequential treatment with the cholera and yellow fever nosodes and saw the child again 3 months later. What a change! The boy still had quite a temperament, but at least I was now dealing with a normal good-natured child. The rest of the treatment comprised of the nosodes for smallpox and the other usual childhood vaccinations, punctuated by the equally classic and common colds of elimination. But the diabolical character of gratuitous violence never returned.

It seems to me that the psyche is always affected by these violent exotic poisons, but the body fares little better. In October 1980 I received a visit from Mme Lily L, a charming young woman whose mother was Congolese. She came to see me because she was no longer able to stand the rigours of our climate. Although she had been living in Switzerland since the age of 15, each winter she was incapacitated for weeks owing to frequent bouts of bronchitis and bronchopneumonia. Being intelligent, she had understood what the treatment invariably proposed by all the doctors consulted was really worth; the everlasting antibiotics had only managed to destroy what little health she had left. Ever since her last 'vigorous' (this was the term used) course of treatment she had become a mere shadow of herself. At our first encounter she had a miserable and incessant little cough bringing up yellowish and viscous spittle; her nasal cavities were blocked with purulent glairs and her digestive system was completely out of order. At the ohmmetric test, all the meridians were very clearly affected. This ill-omened unanimity pointed to the extreme gravity of the situation. After another few years of the treatment she was receiving, a cancer, leukaemia or incurable depression would occur.

I started the treatment with a certain scepticism by helping the emunctory systems (the sanitation department) eliminate my colleagues' chemicals. I followed this with the typhoid nosode in November and yellow fever in December. My patient suffered extreme exhaustion following this correction, and her constipation was at its worst, but she only had one flu all winter! I saw her again in May, and the meridians were a little better but she still had a way to go. Next I attacked the terrible cholera, the last obstacle to their full opening, and had to intervene another five times in 1981 and six times in 1982 to achieve a definitive balance. I saw her again in April 1983, and the three previous winters had all passed without incident, the constipation was gone and the energetic balance was perfect. Mme L no longer needs to fear the return of her bronchitis attacks; she is cured.

I didn't choose these two examples of tropical pathology by accident. One shows a character deterioration and the other a physical debility that can both be attributed to these foreign toxins. I will let you imagine the misery of these lives if homoeopathy hadn't re-established their harmony.

And now I would like to invite you to a small exercise in honest reasoning. Imagine the hundreds of millions of human beings that populate the Third World. Do you realize that these people carry the living germs of these illnesses or their toxins, and many others as well? Do you think it is easy to work in tropical conditions when one's energetic balance has been lost since infancy? Our Western experts, worn out and useless after a stay of a few years, know something about this!

Why is so much going wrong in the under-developed countries? Why do efforts at help always fail? The most knowledgeable economists in the world can find no remedy for the growing misery of the Third World. The white man brings his brothers wheat, fertilizer, machines of all kinds, cannons, drugs, dollars and even the Bible and Karl Marx. But none of these 'gifts' give back to a man the most precious gift he could have: the perfect balance of his vital energy.

I don't think there are many people in the Third World who enjoy this harmony, since it is evident that in addition to the list of troublemakers that we have in our world can be added the inevitable tropical toxins whose importance you have just been able to measure. Until such time as the nosodic cleansing has purified humankind, it is futile to continue the struggle against underdevelopment. Before attacking the structures it is necessary to change people. The evolution towards total degradation is inevitable if the responsible governments do not finally turn towards Real Medicine.

THIRTEEN

BCG and the French malaise

Entire continents slip inexorably towards underdevelopment because their leaders attempt to modify political and economic structures instead of changing people. Seen from my tiny country, this world-wide drama seems so far away that the probability of a similar misadventure on our own soil appears remote to say the least. Yet over the last few years, and more specifically since World War II, attentive observers can study the terrible phenomenon nearby, indeed right next door.

It is evident that France, unless it comes to grips with itself, is on a slippery slope that will lead it to join the group of underdeveloped nations in the next century. This peremptory assertion will have my French readers howling in indignation, if any can be found who are willing to continue reading after this public affront! Unfortunately the signs of this slow decadence are overwhelming, and each time I return from France I have a heavy heart at the thought of seeing the civilization that taught me how to speak sink into greyness.

Is my criticism open to question? Of course it is. I don't have the skills to evaluate the socioeconomic capabilities of this neighbour, nor to judge accurately the value of its industrial and financial potential. These considerations don't interest me. They are no more representative of the real health of a nation than is the gross national product.

No, the signs to which I point are much more subtle. It takes a clinical eye to discern them, not the cold reasoning of a technocrat. Like the first discolorations of leprosy, they are barely perceptible. But when a doctor's suspicions have been awakened the possibility of illness cannot be ignored. It is then essential to be wide awake and not make a wrong diagnosis.

The range of symptoms that alerted me is very wide. Those of you who know and appreciate France have certainly detected some of them yourselves. Here, in no particular order, are a few.

Every year the welcome given to foreigners loses some of its spontaneity. The porter, taxi-driver, waiter, policeman and caretaker are not as good-natured as they once were. The saleslady and usherette are sour faced. The spontaneous kindness of '*la douce France*' is gone. People are tense, their faces sad and strained, their smiles rare. Politeness, once a national virtue, is undoubtedly no longer taught to children.

Even elegance is disappearing. The pretty women one sees walking along the boulevards have Nordic accents. Abroad, Parisian chic no longer makes much of an effect. In certain sophisticated cosmopolitan receptions French women stand apart: they look 'provincial'!

In Paris the plays that are witty or amusing are Anglo-Saxon. Literature is uninspired. Television is no better, dominated by imported programmes and political invective. The inaneness of many French radio programmes is known throughout the French-speaking world; even the language, once so beautiful, is becoming increasingly vulgar.

What has happened to the good taste of the French? Everyday objects have taken on an international uniformity of aspect. Modern design is Scandinavian, Italian or American. French architects are as mediocre as ours and no longer capable of giving us lessons in style, even in civil engineering. Yes, even the highways, tunnels and dams seem to be more graceful in Switzerland …

But let us put these details aside and turn to the essential. What has happened to the famous French intelligence and clear-mindedness, the traditional critical spirit and renowned common sense? How is it that the French, a people so enamoured of freedom and individual liberties that they invented *the* revolution, have become little more than a nation of docile sheep? This current decline is a visible consequence of the infamous '*mal français*' – the French malaise – that has troubled the most reputed analysts, none of whom has succeeded in diagnosing this '*mal*' correctly. And yet the French malaise can be summed up in three letters: BCG.

I am not joking. In fact I have never been more serious. The BCG is the vaccination that the French pride themselves with having invented for the protection of humanity from tuberculosis. Unfortunately this wonderful invention is little more than a poisoned chalice. Let me enlighten you further.

First of all, what do these letters represent? B stands for bacillus, or germ; C and G are the initials of the two inventors of the vaccine. (I shall refrain from giving their names in full; they have done too much harm to France and many other countries as well.)

In the 1920s C and G were employees of the Institut Pasteur in Paris. The substance of their work can be found in a propagandist book entitled *Preventive Vaccination against Tuberculosis with BCG*. The few pages that I remember made a mockery of scientific thought, not to mention simple logic and good sense. It is in fact possible to speak of a very serious breach of intellectual integrity. And we doctors have swallowed this nonsense without a squeak. Why didn't we heed the warning of Dr Paul Chavanon? In his book *Bacteriological War Has Started*, published with urgency in Paris in 1950, this eminent French homoeopath sounded the alarm and revealed the machinations of a devilish plot. Because a plot there was!

The launching of the BCG vaccine was a model of economic gangsterism, a gigantic dishonest commercial operation. Nothing is missing from the scenario: an eccentric inventor, falsified laboratory experiments, a pseudo-scientific varnish, garbled statistics, shameless publicity, the purchased support of powerful magnates, and, the final masterly touch, a 'free' product ... financed by the taxpayer!

For the French public, unfortunately used to scandals, none of this is very uncommon. But what really sets the BCG story apart is the heights of machiavellism that it reaches. For Chavanon reveals that the 20 or so families that hold hostage the nation's health – i.e. its teaching, its laboratories, its temples ... and its commerce – succeeded in 1949 in having the French government hurriedly vote to make the BCG vaccination compulsory. Since that black year not one French person has escaped this fatal toxin, the stealthy agent of that mysterious ailment – the French malaise – which has brought one of the most brilliant civilizations of the Western world to its knees. Dr Chavanon's worst forecasts have become a reality. I am not going to reproduce here the prophetic pages where, with his inimitable flair, this great doctor predicted the worst. Instead, 36 years later, I shall simply present the facts as seen in the light of Real Medicine.

INFANT DEATHS

Let me remind you of something I said earlier. Any vaccination is a shock, a serious shake-up of our delicate energetic balance. The shock can be fatal if a child is vaccinated in the first days of life and if the constitution has certain deficiencies. Since the deaths first exposed by Chavanon and numerous other, objective observers, the list of fatalities has increased by thousands. But no one worries about them since nobody is told. When a bus drives off a mountain road, with 40 schoolchildren on board, the tragedy inevitably makes the front page of the newspapers. The hundreds of children killed each year by the BCG vaccine remain anonymous. This minor inconvenience must be hushed up at all costs; otherwise the Institut Pasteur's goose that lays the golden egg might end up as soup stock! On no account must the medical profession be informed. Disinformation starts with compartmentalization and secrecy. It is the same in Switzerland for the numerous lethal specialities of our powerful pharmaceutical industry, whose victims we are only just starting to count.

Nevertheless any doctor not totally cut off in his ivory tower has heard from his patients at least once of the 'unexplained' death of a newborn infant shortly after a BCG vaccination. Or perhaps he has been a direct witness, if not the cause himself. Multiply this drama by the number of doctors in France and you can begin to get an idea of the magnitude of the disaster. (To this must be added the observations of all the foreign doctors as well.)

I have similar testimony to present, even though this sad reality is considerably rarer in my own country. (In 1949 we rejected overwhelmingly the introduction of compulsory tuberculosis skin tests by a three to one majority. There was no question of imposing the BCG vaccination on the Swiss!) In 1983 I had a visit from the parents of an 8-year-old boy who since birth had suffered from chronic bronchitis that did not respond to any form of treatment. (I shall withhold his name to avoid bringing back painful memories.) I explained to his parents, as at every initial consultation, the principles of my sequential therapy including, of course, any vaccinations. It was quickly apparent that the child's health had been severely compromised from birth following a BCG inoculation when he was only 2 days old. His brother and sister, who had been just as hastily vaccinated at birth, were also chronically ill despite a simple life in the country and a healthy diet. I explained to the parents that a vaccination given suddenly and without preparation to a fragile constitution is a destabilizing shock. They readily accepted this notion. I stated that it seemed to me to be extremely dangerous to inoculate an unweaned infant with BCG, and that hundreds of children had been killed in this manner. A tense and long silence followed this statement. A sudden realization had come to these good people. The mother wiped away a tear and I learned with dismay that a year earlier they had lost a robust and healthy baby just 1 week after this vaccination. The doctors had formulated a classic diagnosis of sudden 'viral encephalitis'. Naturally, no autopsy was proposed.

The truth is disturbing. Every time you hear of the tragic death of an infant, carried off in the first weeks of life by 'viral meningitis', you have the right to suspect that BCG is at work, even if the autopsy confirms a viral diagnosis. My wife lived through this tragedy in a major Swiss hospital where she worked. The autopsy of the child revealed the tubercular nature of the 'viral' meningitis following a BCG inoculation, but all the assistants and nurses had received very clear instructions to say nothing or risk terrible consequences. As with all secret societies, the law of silence is absolute among doctors!

Faced with a knowledgeable public, the medical profession can no longer deny that an early BCG shock is capable of killing. It is accepted as a general and faraway eventuality, but the tone changes when reality presents a concrete case. In front of the body of a newborn child, the doctor denies any involvement and hides the truth with the help of his colleagues. This ignoble attitude degrades and dishonours our profession. Furthermore, it distorts scientific information and misleads the honest student, who, once a doctor, will also vaccinate in good faith, completely unaware of the tremendous risk to infants. I too, at the beginning of my career, was unaware of this indiscriminate slaughter and had vaccinated schoolchildren, luckily older and less vulnerable.

But I was ignorant of other things as well. I did not realize that the BCG vaccine could bring about worse things than death. Yes, blessed is the soul that takes wing again so soon after birth; the pain remains for the parents. But what can be said for those crippled lives that society hastens to hide in specialized institutions? Before my accession to Real Medicine, the disjointed puppet-like bodies of cerebral–motor victims filled me with compassion. Since then that feeling has often been replaced by one of indignation. Cerebral–motor victims, like many others who bear congenital defects, owe their sad condition to the main cause of all illnesses: an imbalance of vital energy. This is naturally the consequence of a shock: genetic, prenatal or postnatal.

If the shock is too violent, life is not possible. The egg is not fertilized, or the fetus is not capable of further development, the child is stillborn or dies shortly after birth. If the shock is better withstood, the egg develops but is defective. The same is true of the fetus or the newborn child.

You now know enough to be able to imagine the role played by the BCG vaccination. At the time of writing (1984), it was at the top of the list of traumatisms inflicted on newly born children in the maternity wards, way ahead of smallpox vaccinations or other 'strong' interventions. Why this sad precedence when French law has never imposed that the vaccination occur before the age of 6 years? Because certain doctors have allowed themselves to be convinced by the manufacturer's propaganda that early tuberculosis inoculation is the most effective method of fighting the disease. These doctors are all the more insistent where new mothers are concerned if there is a family history of the illness. But more often than not they impose the vaccinal shock without the knowledge of the parents, in violation of the most elementary individual rights. This is why, of all the destabilizing events that threaten the vital balance of a newborn child, BCG is the one that appears most frequently in the dock.

But what does such a shock do in the first days of a life? As we have seen, it can kill. If the constitution is less specifically vulnerable to tuberculosis – that is, if it is not very 'tuberculinous' – the vaccination will not kill, but can create a lifelong infirmity. Of course, I am not saying that all cerebral–motor victims owe their condition to this vaccine, nor that all BCG vaccinations cause this infirmity, but it happens that the few cases of this kind that I have treated had all received this vaccination shortly after birth. Curiously, other homoeopathic colleagues with whom I have shared these thoughts have noticed the same thing. I do not have enough space here to give you in full the sad anamnesis of one or another of these poor children. But it is essential that I point out one very troubling fact that considerably reinforces the presumption of BCG's harmful nature, and that provides overwhelming proof of its considerable impact on the cerebral sphere. This proof is provided by the spectacular improvement of all the neuromotor functions immediately following the prescription of the vaccinal nosode. We can recall the case of little Mathias, who was saved from a future as an invalid by the correct isotherapeutic sequence. In his case the critical motor progress occurred only after the BCG had been erased.

Here homoeopathic treatment takes on an additional value, unavailable to chemotherapy: that of hope rekindled by the tiniest new spark of vital energy. The hope is even more justified if the imbalance is not too pronounced or too deeply anchored in the past. If the patient comes to consult the doctor in time, as soon as the first signs of mental retardation have been noticed, it is not impossible to hope for the complete recovery that is not accessible to allopathic doctors and their drugs.

The tubercular BCG shock is strong enough to kill or forever debilitate the fragile little being. If the child is more robust or a little older, he will escape this awful fate, particularly if the paediatrician gives him enough time to recover his balance before giving another vaccination. But don't think that he's out of danger. Remember, a vaccination is always a shock, and the destabilizing tubercular shock can have after-effects leading to chronic illness and the poisoning of a whole life. Owing to the multiple forms of its long-term consequences, the BCG vaccination is without question the champion of all destabilizers. It subdues the nervous system. It dominates digestive pathology. It ravages pulmonary functions. It is a goldmine for the ENT specialist. It oppresses the osteoarticular system. It blemishes the skin. It causes allergies to flourish. It poisons the urogenital system.

For each of these categories here are a few thoughts, sometimes accompanied by examples from my practice, summarized as succinctly as possible. At the end of the list I will return to the long-term psychological effects of this vaccination, which to my mind are the justification for the title of this chapter. But first, let us begin with the following, less speculative considerations.

DIGESTIVE PATHOLOGY

BCG dominates digestive pathology. This is not surprising since tuberculosis is above all an illness of the intestinal flora like its cousin, leprosy. Even in its pulmonary, osseous, renal or meningeal forms, the virulence of the germ that spreads this disease requires a prior collapse of the intestinal ecology.

Most Western doctors are unaware of this traditional Eastern concept, but the physiologists who are preparing the scientific truths of the 21st century already suspect some kind of subtle relationship linking congenital predispositions, digestive flora, nutrition and the energetic Large Intestine–Lung connection that is well known to acupuncturists. I don't want to back up these statements with scholarly demonstrations, since that is not the purpose of a book destined to a broad public. My goal is rather to provide information and to anchor a conviction through example rather than through theory. Here then is what I observe in my day to day experience.

I have lost count of the number of children who complain of various digestive reactions after receiving the BCG nosode in my therapeutic sequence. Since my nosode is immaterial (a placebo according to the faculty), one has to admit that the very real stomach ache following its ingestion is the expression of the organism's reaction to this coded impulse. What is extraordinary is that this liberating shock is usually sufficient to cure definitively those awful chronic stomach aches that make little children cry and their doctors despair. Every paediatrician has been confronted more than once with this irritating problem. The primary symptom of this commonplace scene is eloquent in its simplicity: the child points his finger at his navel; that's where it hurts, right there in the middle of the stomach.

The number of examinations can be increased and gastro-intestinal specialists can be consulted, but additional clues will be few and treatments disappointing. The compassionate paediatricians will prescribe spasmolytics offering temporary relief. The more intelligent ones will quickly recognize the futility of their efforts and prescribe nothing further. The more pedantic will drug these poor children with tranquillizers. Each of these approaches results in the same decision for the parents: they lose confidence in the doctor and seek help elsewhere.

The charlatans are not much more successful. But the honest practitioners of natural techniques can provide tremendous relief. Foot massage, lymphatic draining, auricular therapy, acupuncture and all the 'gentle' medicines are preferable to the habitual response of my colleagues, which is to add to the problem through medicinal intoxication. But if the BCG is responsible for the problem, only its nosode will correctly erase the energetic distortion and cure the patient. Because they have not learned the lessons of isopathy, most traditional homoeopaths also fail in their interminable treatments and are jealous of the success of informed radiesthesists who quickly find the correct nosode and are able to heal.

I do not intend to imply by this analysis that all stomach aches can be attributed to BCG. This common symptom also occurs in non-vaccinated children. But it is so frequently present as the sign of an artificial tubercular disorder that I had to mention it first. Other frequently voiced complaints that can be attributed to the vaccine are swelling, exaggerated fermentation, painful intestinal colic, chronic constipation and diarrhoea. It is really wonderful for the doctor to be able to free the patient from these things in a few days when the time has come to give the nosode. The medical act is so simple! I usually have to go up to the 10,000th Korsakovian potency after what is often a prudent and slow approach. It can sometimes take a whole month of little nudges before giving the necessary shock, but the liberating reaction always follows, weak or powerful. After a few hours of painful cramps – at the worst – or a few days of flu-like intestinal trouble, the rebellious symptoms completely disappear for good.

PULMONARY DISORDERS

BCG ravages the pulmonary system. This is obvious. Without being a doctor anyone can understand that a vaccination that claims to protect us from pulmonary tuberculosis entails the risk – inherent to the mission – of inducing a pulmonary symptomatology. It is part of the very nature of its shock wave, its amplitude and frequency.

Here again, I will not bore you with theoretical considerations.

The abundance of blatant cases of pathological pulmonary reactivation following a BCG detoxification is adequate to prove the close correlation between the vaccinal toxin and the observed problems. In this case also, the correct administration of the nosode is enough to erase these troubles, as if by a magic wand. Begone bronchitis and broncho-pneumonia! Disappear chronic cough, colds, wheezing and bronchitis, which ruin our winters! And germs and viruses fall back. Let our revived defences take over the operations, and freed from its tubercular yoke, the immunological counter-attack deploys itself in a new and more appropriate way. Recovery is quickly obtained.

But be careful! Avoid the precipitation of Mme L who came to see me for her little 8-year-old Josiane who had become an invalid following a BCG injection 10 days after a DiTePer vaccination. The poor child had been coughing for 8 months as if she was going to die when her parents finally decided to change doctors. I easily found the guilty party and began the isosequential treatment. When I reached BCG, a key episode, I pushed the dose of its nosode up to XMK and unleashed an enormous pulmonary reaction with a high fever. The mother hadn't given the copper–gold–silver catalyst that I had prescribed beforehand to stimulate the defences and diminish the expected reaction.

Panicked, the mother went back to her previous paediatrician. He took a blood sample, X-rayed the lungs, diagnosed broncho-pneumonia and applied the logic he had learned: illness equals infection plus inflammation. The treatment? None other than the ever-present reflex of antibiotics and anti-inflammatories: paracetamol for the inflammation and our old friend Clamoxyl for the unidentified germ.

Naturally Mme L didn't admit to her ex-doctor that she had taken the child to a homoeopath. He inevitably would have made fun of her and of me and wouldn't have understood what was happening to the child anyway. Allopathic doctors are completely unaware of the classic and very beneficial homoeopathic reactional aggravation, and when confronted with it by chance tend to mistake it for a real worsening of the ailment.

Following this mishap, I had first to repair the chemical damage, losing 10 days to drain the liver and kidneys and to repeat the last dose of the nosode, which had not had time to take effect. The outcome was rapid and simple. Once the BCG barrier had been overcome the cough stopped and Josiane's health returned. The mother got off with a passing fright, the necessary psychological ransom for someone with one foot in the old and one in the new method of medical practice. This type of behaviour can result in the failure of a treatment if the patient lacks sufficient courage. But most of the time the initial uncertainty evolves towards an increasing assurance, since nothing is more invigorating than seeing the realization of the doctor's most optimistic predictions.

ENT DISORDERS

BCG is a goldmine for ear, nose and throat specialists. This small area in which these colleagues exercise their art is of major importance in infant morbidity. It is certain that the vast majority of childhood visits to the doctor are prompted by an acute or chronic inflammation of the rhinopharynx or middle ear. Parents very quickly diagnose by themselves an inflammation of the throat or otitis, and they can be roughly grouped in three categories.

The confirmed optimists put themselves in the hands of nature and consult their doctor only in extremely serious cases. The worriers and those who obediently follow the official doctrine readily accept the only proposed treatment: chemical intoxication. But growing numbers of thoughtful people no longer allow themselves to be taken in. More mentally alert than the doctors, these enlightened parents are able to see beyond the technical jargon and recognize behind it the real content of this academic language: an unbelievable poverty of intellect. They now keep their ears open ('listen to unfounded rumours', according to the doctors), observe the results obtained by energetic (ie non-material) techniques and they make comparisons. It doesn't take long for them to admit unreservedly the value of Real Medicine and they quickly become enthusiastic followers.

And you, dear reader, to which camp do you belong? If you are a partisan of a natural method, you take care of your children's bad throats yourselves and run a certain risk, albeit minimal. If you opt for the faculty, you run to the paediatrician with every cold and accept a medicinal intoxication. The risk of short-term complications is smaller, but you are taking out a mortgage with a higher, deferred repayment. And if instead you open your eyes to the truth, you accept the artificial risk of a simulated aggravation while maintaining the integrity of your child's fundamental health.

These three tendencies can be best illustrated by a study of nose and throat pathology. In the past, throat inflammations were not treated, heart and kidney complications were frequent and child mortality decimated families. Since Alexander Fleming, treatments have become 'powerful', and doctors no longer mourn so many victims. All year round, the same scenes repeat themselves millions of times over throughout the civilized world. The most classical scenario is the following:

A child is born, the family celebrates, the baby grows and thrives normally. Then comes the day for his presentation in the Temple – that is, at the altar of Science. The child receives his ritual mark ... and the troubles begin. Most of the time the over-vaccination results only in passing colds and a few shivers. At least for the first generation of those vaccinated. But for each of the following generations the genetic pollution is progressively, slowly reinforced, as with chemical pollution in the food chain. The individual constitution is undermined. The vital energy no longer resonates as it wishes and loses its balance like a tightrope walker deprived of his pole. Disaster can now occur at the drop of a hat. The shock can come from any virus at all, identified or not. Thousands of strains are now known, and there are probably millions just waiting for the opportunity to multiply now that tons of antibiotics have been dumped on the planet and destroyed the bacteriological ecosystems of millennia.

These conquering germs are everywhere: in the air, the water, on every object and surface, on the skin. Children cannot be brought up in the totally antiseptic environment of a laboratory. They have to learn to live with these dangerous companions, to whom they must none the less refuse access to their internal environment. This isn't easy since the citadel of our physical bodies offers a gaping hole: the upper aerodigestive crossroad: the mouth, nose and linked tracts. The ENT area is the preferred entry point for bacteriological invasion. You can easily imagine why so many conflicts start with the noisy effervescence of its outposts.

And so the virus boldly enters the stronghold. The vital energy that has been imbalanced by overvaccination can no longer bolster the defence mechanisms. Something is lacking in the high command and the entire weight of defence rests with the autonomy of isolated pockets of resistance. Most important among these are the tonsils, the advance bastions of the support system. Scorned until recently, they are full of near-electronic sensory systems and play a determining role in immune guidance. But they still can't replace an army, and the most sophisticated system is barely good enough for a parade if the high command isn't there.

Throat inflammation or common pharyngitis is the outcome. Under the repeated assaults of the attackers, the inflammation often becomes chronic and home remedies are no longer good enough. The paediatrician is consulted and prescribes the usual treatment. An antibiotic calms the first attack, and maybe even the next few, but it doesn't prevent recurrence. Since the doctor blindly believes in Pasteur's theory of germs, he attributes these failures to the appearance of bacterial resistance. Therefore the strength and diversity of the antibiotics used has to be increased, and big pharmaceutical companies are only too happy to offer their voluntary sales force evermore new all-purpose or specialized antibiotics. Through their publicity they convince naive doctors that a wide-ranging antibiotic is the absolute weapon for such and such an infection or problem. The trusting doctors prescribe the new remedy, which works for a while, but the return of the illness soon dashes their hopes. Faced with the apparent permanence of the ailment and pressed by the anxious parents, the paediatrician must save face. Their way out is always at hand: to call in a specialist to help.

And what do specialists do? Are they any better armed than their colleagues? The chemical weapons are the same. They have only one other way out: surgery. Tonsils are the designated victim. For a long time, and by tens of millions, they have been feeding the unsteady finances of clinics and hospitals while at the same time guaranteeing a comfortable income to those colleagues who are gifted with their hands. This operation is often effective and brings back an appearance of health, but it never restores the child's lost energetic balance. Most of the time it suppresses an entire range of symptoms while establishing another scoreboard elsewhere. There are countless cases of chronic and incurable laryngitis and bronchitis that have been definitively established following a tonsillectomy. But ENT specialists aren't concerned about this; beyond the edge of their little preserve other specialists will be interested by this new pathology.

The parents go to see the internist, the physiologist, the allergy specialist and even the psychiatrist, all to no avail. As long as the destabilizing sequence has not been identified and corrected, the chronic illness triumphs. You may be wondering why I bring up this stream of rhinopharyngeal episodes in a chapter about the French malaise. It is because the BCG vaccination is far and away the most traumatizing event of infancy, way ahead of other vaccinations, anaesthesia and many commotions. And since the ENT area is the first window of childhood illnesses, it is only natural that I should point out the principal guilty party.

The French malaise brings wealth to the specialists and Real Medicine ruins them! I won't hide the fact that I spend most of my time correcting the disturbed balance of dozens of children with colds and sore throats. As soon as the corrective sequence has been deployed, harmony quickly returns and my other colleagues are rarely visited. Among the hundred or so children that I see every year for the first time, I rarely ask that more than two or three have their tonsils out. And now I also send them to a specialist who is fully aware of energetic realities so that the parents are protected from the sarcastic comments of badly informed half-doctors. In the vast majority of cases sequential therapy works miracles, particularly if the constitution is flexible and reacts well to my coded input. The throat inflammations become infrequent and from then on react to the simple little remedies of traditional homoeopathy.

But there is another advantage, which I must emphasize. I almost never see acute cases of appendicitis any more! This statement may seem incredible if you do not see the logical link between BCG, the tonsils and the appendix. It is nevertheless real, and can be proven very simply. Overvaccination destabilizes the child's vital energy, and BCG is the finishing touch weakening the first line of defence: the lymphatic system of the aerodigestive crossroad. The tonsils are wrongly considered as responsible and hence removed. The defences then organize themselves along a second strategic line: the lymphatic system of the intestinal tract. The appendix was very appropriately recognized by the anatomists of the last century as 'the tonsils of the stomach', and has yet to reveal all its secrets. Like the tonsils, it plays a considerable role in immunological performance, and certainly takes over from the tonsils in certain defensive functions. But it too can be exhausted by the failure of the first filters, giving rise to acute appendicitis and requiring an urgent operation!

I often play the following detective's game. Each time the anamnesis of a new patient reveals that he or she has been operated for appendicitis, I dig a little deeper and discover that the tonsils were removed a few years earlier. This observation is too frequent to be pure chance. Three times out of four, if the doctor assumes that this has been the case he will be proven correct. Given the millions of urgent appendix operations throughout the world, one can only hope for a rapid extension of Real Medicine.

OSTEOARTICULAR PROBLEMS

The BCG also oppresses the osteoarticular system. I won't launch into useless theoretical explanations since I think by now you have understood the down-to-earth approach of this book. Here again, examples are better than speculation.

On 29 November 1979 I had a visit from Christophe M, aged 7 years. In July he had suddenly started complaining of vague articular pains, which rapidly spread to the elbows and knees making any movement painful. The terrible diagnosis had fallen like a guillotine dropping: the child was suffering from acute articular rheumatism. The doctor had only two pitiful weapons to offer: antibiotics and anti-inflammatory drugs. Cortisone was prescribed and things seemed to improve, but not for long. Penicillin at very high doses was administered. A renowned specialist was consulted and was even less reassuring: Christophe was condemned to take penicillin for the next 10 years! The parents, better informed than the doctors, knew that an alternative solution existed and came to see me.

The child's anamnesis was quickly laid out. He had never been ill before and had not had any of the usual childhood illnesses. The only shocks to be found were the usual vaccinations: DTPP in 1972, smallpox in 1973 and BCG four months later. I started the treatment by eliminating the penicillin and the cortisone. The child seemed better but was still in pain. Logically, I should then have continued with the isotherapeutic sequence of the vaccinations, particularly since the meridians all seemed perfectly balanced on the ohmmeter. But between 1979 and 1973 there were a few suspiciously empty years which I couldn't risk skipping just in case the key to the problem was to be found there by accident. My questioning became more pointed and I learned that a neighbour's child had recently come down with a strong case of scarlet fever. The mother claimed that Christophe had not caught the illness, but my pendulum reacted strongly to the corresponding nosode. Knowing the critical role played by the streptococcus in rheumatism, I was jubilant, and ordered a high potency of Scarlatinum for early January. The child developed a fever with vomiting 2 days later, but still didn't recover. I managed to find mumps that had also gone unnoticed, and corrected the traces in February. The child had improved, but his joints were still swollen. In mid March I returned to the logical sequence and was able to attack the BCG of 1973.

Immediately after taking the nosode, a miracle occurred. All the joints became swollen and were then freed over the following days. Christophe was cured. In April I erased the smallpox, in May the DTPP, and throughout 1981 I corrected the constitution. Signs of relapse in the right elbow were stopped instantly in May 1984 with three doses of Ledum and two of Calcarea fluorica. Since 1979 the boy has not received any chemicals and is doing very well without them. I have saved him from 10 years of daily antibiotic treatment and perhaps even given him the gift of a few more years of life.

Who can say how many artificial 'rheumatics' have prematurely become invalids because of the BCG vaccination? No one really knows, and only adepts of isopathic therapy can even make an approximate guess. Like me they sometimes set off a terrible crisis of rheumatism with the nosode, thus proving its guilty role in so many hidden problems.

But the main point of this criticism is the message of hope brought by these recoveries. If the energetic distortion created by this poison is correctly eliminated by the nosode, the osteoarticular patient can rapidly be cured of his chronic problems, just like those who suffer from throat inflammation, bronchitis or chronic digestive problems.

DERMATOLOGICAL PROBLEMS AND ALLERGIES

BCG is also unequalled in creating dermatological problems. I have lost count of the hundreds of children whose parents have asked me to remove their multiple spots, rashes and itches. After a few visits to the dermatologist they quickly get tired of the unique treatment proposed – efficacious, that is for sure, since almost all modern ointments contain cortisone derivatives, but perfectly useless – and harmful – in the long term. Informed parents no longer accept the clever labels given to the illness. They would rather listen to the 'gossip' passed on by the cleaning lady and put themselves in the hands of gentler techniques. Acupuncture, clay and cabbage leaves are wonderful, but only isotherapy will smooth the skin if it is BCG that has brought on the ruin of a weakened constitution. Its hold on the evacuating mechanisms of the skin is amazingly strong.

In the summer of 1980 I saw Sandra P, aged 6 years, whose mother undressed her very slowly in my presence. On the left half of the thorax was an enormous infected skin wound, swollen and painful. The dermatologist consulted before me had prescribed antibiotic and anti-inflammatory ointment (always the same reflex!) without even listening to the mother's opinion. Yet she had clearly told him that the problem appeared shortly following the patch-test for tuberculosis used by all school doctors. What the specialist took to be a common microbial infection was really an enormous reaction to the tubercular ointment. The tuberculin used for this test is the same as BCG but much more diluted. If a tiny fraction of this poison is enough to create such terrible damage, you can imagine how virulent a full BCG vaccination must be! And I am not thinking here of physical scars, like the huge purulent crater that a paediatrician had managed to carve into the thigh of Alexandra C, the daughter of a friend who came seeking help from me in the hope of repair. I am referring instead to the despairing eczemas that can destroy an entire life through the size of the wounds and the dreadful ferocity of the itching they incur.

Yes, BCG literally inflames allergies. Incurable skin diseases are often just the painful evidence of that modern pathology, the allergy. For once the two warring sisters, allopathy and homoeopathy, agree in their recognition of its growing importance. Both recognize the notion of allergic heredity, but this is where the agreement stops. For the allopathic doctors, chronic allergic illness is treated with chemical antiallergenic means. Since failure is the rule in the long run, desensitizing therapy is increasingly being used. Without realizing it doctors have come a little closer to homoeopathic reasoning, but they quickly encounter the same disappointment. Their treatment is lacking the essential element: the dematerialization/ potentization which alone has the ability to flirt with Life.

These allopathic inventions may not have the capacity to harmonize vital energy, but they unfortunately do have the dangerous ability to destroy it. It is always easier to break a piece of fine china than it is to glue it back together. In allergic illnesses, as in any chronic illness, the iatrogenic shock that is most capable of 'breaking' something is once again BCG.

Here is an example of its hidden role in the most tenacious skin problem and also the toughest of allergies, eczema. Once again, I do not want to imply that BCG was the cause of the illness. It is merely the most subtle complicating factor combined with others to create a kind of suffocating etheric stickiness which causes the imbalance.

When young Boris S's parents (from Crans-sur-Sierre) brought him to see me, I was shown the most incredible case of eczema of my career. The poor child emerging from his bandages was one vast purulent wound from head to toe. Only the sad eyes that could be discerned through his sticky lashes contained a sign of life's beauty. I couldn't find a healthy piece of skin on which to place my electrodes, but never mind! An ohmmeter was hardly needed to diagnose the extent of his energetic imbalance. The anamnesis gave me the two key elements for evaluation of the problem. First of all, his hereditary allergic background was confirmed. Secondly, I obtained the complete sequence of all major shocks. Since the child was only a year old, the list was short: BCG at 2 months then three DTPPs. I began by neutralizing these two events with their respective nosodes in September and November. I saw the child again in December. The improvement had been spectacular following the BCG. The child no longer had to be entirely rebandaged every day, and hope had returned. I then applied myself to the long work on the hereditary situation, which took 2 years. Today Boris can rest assured that he will not have to suffer the same torments as his father who was afflicted in this way up to the age of 20. The eczema has been gone since 1982. Will it come back? No one can know, but one thing is certain: no treatment would have been able to succeed if I had not first erased the trace of the French ailment.

In asthma and hayfever the negative impact of BCG is every bit as critical since it feeds all the visible manifestations of the same constitutional defect. I have never been able to cure a vaccinated person's asthma without first removing the etheric deformation left by the injected tuberculin. The day that allergists understand this truth they will be able to abandon their useless and fastidious desensitizing cures to the great benefit of the patients and their wallets.

UROGENTIAL PROBLEMS

BCG also poisons the urogenital system. You now know my reasoning: tuberculosis attacks the lungs, the intestines, the bones, the skin, and so on. The tuberculin of its vaccine therefore ravages the same targets. Since the illness also destroys the kidneys, there is no reason to think that the tuberculin wouldn't do the same thing. This additional misdeed of BCG is less well known, but is none the less very real. The lack of documented observations is due strictly to the rarity of kidney pathology. For every hundred children that I see with coughs and colds, I perhaps see only three or four with kidney or bladder problems. But I apply the same suspicious questioning to everyone, and am therefore not surprised to find BCG once again at the top of the list of destabilizing shocks.

When I saw Marianne G, aged 9 years, (from La Tour-de-Peilz) she had been suffering for a year from chronic cystitis (*Escherichia coli*). Her doctor had unsuccessfully tried the full range of antibiotics, but the urine remained infected. Maintaining confidence for over a year is no longer acceptable for an informed public. Compared with homoeopathy, it is official medicine that suddenly has the look of charlatanism. The child was brought to me in April 1983. The disturbing sequence was totally iatrogenic, ending up with BCG injected in November 1979. After repairing the multiple chemical injuries inflicted by the previous doctor, I attacked the energetic treatment on the BCG nosode at the outset. The reaction was immediate: a strong case of pharyngitis, followed – for the last time – by a strong bacterial discharge in the urine. I saw her again in June, in September and in November. She has never had cystitis again. She is cured.

The real benefit Marianne will have gained from the treatment can never be fully measured. What would have happened to her kidney functions if I had not intervened so soon? Do you think the kidneys can go calmly about their business when the bladder is constantly overworked? Of course not. When a civil war is going on in a country its neighbours are necessarily affected. If the kidney function is altered, the worst is always possible despite all the resources of chemotherapy.

The scenario of a classic complication is fairly simple. Most of the time the family doctor notices the insidious appearance of an arterial hypertension that is uncommon in young people. Sometimes it is the school doctor who is first to ring the alarm bell. Specialists are consulted, and analyses are carried out at great expense, but all in vain. 'Half-doctors' can't find the cause of the illness since they obstinately refuse to accept what is essential. But if the patient sees a 'whole' doctor, such a trifle can be corrected in no time at all. Here is a brief illustration of such a case.

I had a visit from Stephane S (from Peseux) in September 1983 following detection of arterial hypertension at school. At 15/10, the blood pressure was really too high for his 15 years of age. I discovered a common series of morbid and iatrogenic shocks and then began treatment: Morbillinum first, for his measles at the age of 7, then Parotidinum for the attack of mumps at the age of 6. I saw Stephane again in November and the pressure was still at 14/9. I then attacked the next suspect on the list: BCG at age 5. The next examination finally reassured everyone. His blood pressure was down to 11/8 and stable with no medication.

I wanted to cite this example because it points out an essential truth. It is extremely important to start a corrective treatment as quickly as possible. The closer the corrective sequence is to the perturbing sequence, the greater are the chances of recovery. This is even true for an illness that is as totally incurable as chronic arterial hypertension, which official medicine can only help by making it bearable throughout a lifetime.

I have not been as lucky with those patients who came to me 20 years too late. For them, particularly if they had been 'protected' by C and G's discovery, I was not able to remove the old etheric ghosts, and I also had to resign myself to taking care of them with the mediocre medicine of my colleagues.

Tuberculosis often attacks the genital organs as well, particularly with women. There is therefore no reason to be surprised by the impressive number of gynaecological problems that can be observed in the years following the injection of the tuberculin. Here again, I am not accusing BCG as being uniquely responsible for this entire and vast pathology. But young women feel so much better after an isopathic cure that I thought this last gift of Real Medicine was worth mentioning.

CENTRAL NERVOUS SYSTEM DISORDERS

I hope that this somewhat lengthy review may have awakened certain personal memories that might deepen your interest in these new ideas and perhaps encourage you to put them into practice.

Through the first cases evoked at the beginning of the chapter, a brief overview of cerebral–motor infirmities, I tried to draw your attention to the considerable impact that a BCG injection can have on the central nervous system. You certainly also noticed that the flaws I rather fiercely caricatured in the French all belong to the area of higher intelligence, creativity and willpower. This juxtaposition was intentional and designed to better prepare you for the shock of the truth. What I am presently writing is dictated by my intimate and profound conviction, even if for the moment there are no laboratory experiments to confirm the truth of my suppositions. The fact is that an honest doctor has no right to experiment with anyone's life. His only right is to observe.

I believe that what I have observed in all objectivity is profoundly true, even given the enormity of the discovery. The following is what astounds me.

All the therapeutic sequences that I administered to my patients brought about a very clear improvement of their intellectual capacities if they included the BCG nosode. Without this, only a physical improvement occurred. What this means is that BCG alters in a constant and durable manner people's mental capabilities. It introduces an imperceptible defect into the genetic structures that are responsible for intelligence. It creates a new, defective race. When applied by suicidal decree to an entire population, it becomes a national catastrophe, the greatest that France has faced in its entire history.

It is this that is the French malaise.

* * *

The improvement that isotherapy brings to the victims of this disaster is really spectacular. It is the real proof that my suppositions are correct. One slow and stupid child suddenly becomes intelligent following administration of the nosode. Another, severely inhibited, suddenly starts expressing himself. Another, obtuse and unimaginative, suddenly begins writing creative essays. The grades of yet another who was always last in class suddenly improve dramatically. I am amazed by the number of unthought-of successes in school that parents report to me after this French ailment has been erased isosequentially.

And the character changes as well, transformed from irritable and suspicious to gracious and open to the joys of life. Children become reasonable and participate with enthusiasm in the treatment. They are mentally too clever not to recognize the change themselves. Even adults can change personality. I will always remember one obnoxious and blasé Frenchwoman who would come to my consulting rooms to fetch the prescriptions she imposed on me and who became as agreeable and charming as my usual patients after taking the famous nosode.

These prodigious transformations have to be seen to fully appreciate the enormity of the French ailment and the fantastic isotherapeutic power of its nosode. Doctors who have not witnessed these conversions will not be able to accept my revelations. Never mind! It is not for them that I am writing this book. In fact, I would have real trouble trying to explain in scientific terms why BCG degrades both the individual and the race as a whole.

Perhaps esotericists should have their say at this point. They are better than doctors at discerning the subtle relationships that govern all manifestations of Being. Their colourful and extremely poetic language brings us to the heart of the problem. For this terrible daily drama taking place in France, an irrational, analogical explanation prevails over logic.

The BCG tuberculin is a bovine tuberculin. As with smallpox, doctors have never dared to inoculate using the human illness itself. All such experiments have failed. The germ used today comes from cows. And the law has thus imposed on all French people the injection of a proteidic substance of animal origin into the child body of a human being. Vegetarians have maintained for ages that the ingestion of animal flesh gradually introduces the bestiality of the dead animal into the human. Jesus Christ, certainly the greatest doctor of the bimillennary era of Pisces, maintained the same thing in his medical teachings. But we are not speaking here of ingestion. BCG isn't eaten, but injected through the skin. It escapes the control of the skin, that wonderful organ that guards our physical integrity, acting like an emitting and receiving antenna to our brain, and that would never have allowed naturally such an intrusion.

And those two accomplices C and G didn't choose the animal by accident. They chose the cow; this peaceful bovine is slowly but surely becoming the analogical and quasiparental link of the extended family of the French. We are now seeing the appearance of a fourth generation of vaccinated people. What will remain of their once proud national individualism after the seventh generation? Given what is left after three obligatory passages, we can be pretty sure there won't be much. Soon there may be nothing left of the French but a vast herd of bovinized humans.

You think that I am exaggerating? Biologists are now rediscovering the prodigious conceptual and technological advance of knowledgeable alchemists and esoteric philosophers. The bestialization of humanity is in the process of being explained through the progress in genetic research. Computers have familiarized us all with the concept of codes and programming. Our genetic code is not inalterable and the parasitic emanations coming from bioenergetic animal structures might not leave our fragile receptors indifferent and undamaged. No scholar worthy of the name today would ridicule the African sorcerer who inspires young warriors by making them eat a lion's heart.

This highly charged chapter may seem to some excessive, even malicious. I agree it has the harsh tones of an indictment and the acidity of a satirical tract, but it is also an urgent plea that we put an end to our collective mutilation and the further spread of the French malaise. If you don't believe me, read Chavanon, Delarue or the others. In Paris there is a national league for freedom of vaccinations. Contact them and inform yourself. It might then be possible to force the politicians to take the required decision: the banning of BCG.

If something isn't done quickly, this leprosy will contaminate all of Europe. Here, in neighbouring Switzerland, we are already ill. For the past 20 years the Swiss French have lamented the fact that slowly but surely they are being 'colonized' by the Swiss Germans. How can we resist this phenomenon if all the French cantons are afflicted with the French malaise? Our small country serves as an almost experimental demonstration of my hypothesis. Without acknowledging the fact, French Switzerland falls into line with France in medical matters. The local groups for protection against tuberculosis all jumped at the deceptive bait offered by the BCG publicity and the doctors vaccinate wholesale despite the clearly expressed wishes of the population in 1942. They are deceiving the public by claiming that the regression of tuberculosis is due to the introduction of its so-called vaccine. Let them enquire in India where its performance has been so catastrophic that the World Health Organization still has not had the courage to divulge it publicly.

The retreat of tuberculosis in the industrialized nations has nothing to do with medicine, but rather with progress in hygiene, the health of livestock and a general improvement in living standards. In some Anglo-Saxon countries the French vaccine is virtually unknown even though to my knowledge tuberculosis is no more frequent there than in France or Switzerland. The only means available to doctors to fight this terrible illness preventatively are once again homoeopathic. Starting at a very young age the constitution must be fortified to avoid leaving it vulnerable to a bacteriological invasion at a later stage. (The third part of this book will provide more information concerning this fundamental concept of constitutions.) As for BCG, far from protecting its unfortunate beneficiary, it very seriously aggravates the predisposition to catch the illness. I know what I am talking about on the subject as I spent 20 months of my internship in a large mountain sanatorium. The rare incurable cases of tuberculosis that we lost had all been inoculated with the BCG before falling ill!

It is always dangerous to mistake our desires for reality. In the Swiss-German part of our country the general public are less dreamy and more realistic. And they don't like things that come from France, especially in those cantons where the memory of atrocities committed by the armies of the last century lingers on. Therefore, there are fewer people vaccinated, and a less defective race. But I have something even better to recount as experimental proof. This will be my last anecdote.

In 1964 I worked for a few weeks as a health officer on a military review board. In Switzerland the recruiting process involves a short intelligence test including a written composition. The last two districts that I examined were rigorously identical from a demographic standpoint. They had the same race, language, agrarian background, degree of interbreeding and involvement with alcohol. Yet one group's test results were dramatically different, showing a clear intellectual inferiority to the other. Why such a difference? I only realized why many years later when it was my time to encounter Real Medicine. In the 'less intelligent' district all the children were born in the same maternity ward. I learned from the patients whom I later treated and who came from this area that the head doctor of this hospital had been known for ages as an ardent partisan of antitubercular treatments. He had given strict orders – no baby was to leave his clinic without receiving the BCG vaccination, with or without the knowledge of the parents. I don't know whether this man is still alive, but an entire rural area can now thank him for this ironic and incalculable handicap, the most cruel form of degradation – that of the race itself.

FOURTEEN

Childhood illnesses

Future generations will consider overvaccination as one of the most grotesque vagaries in the history of medicine. A day will come when real doctors, at last in large numbers, will affirm as I have that it was the principal element of energetic destabilization in the 20th century, the primary source of all illness.

But doctors are not the only ones responsible for their patients' chronic illnesses. Nature, as we know, is also cruel. She it was who invented the demanding steeplechase of childhood illnesses, this compulsory passage between infancy and adulthood. On that count she is truly pitiless. Depending on how one goes through these childhood illnesses one will later on be a 'sufferer' or healthy.

Clearly a child's vital energy is severely tested during this period of creative expansion. It can even be stated that childhood illness is a shock. Like vaccination, it permanently marks the delicate immaterial skein of our energetic cabling, more or less deeply depending on its intensity. This mark lasts a lifetime. If it is weak, it doesn't exercise a negative influence on the transmission of spatiotemporal vibrations to the lower continuum. Health is sustained. But if it is strong, the reception can be significantly disturbed. The message is garbled, barely comprehensible, as with a badly tuned radio.

In line with popular intuition, homoeopaths long ago noticed that a childhood illness that doesn't 'come out' properly disturbs the organism's reactional abilities. A given child who normally could be steered towards health with a minor vegetal remedy, suddenly needs high potencies of a mineral remedy after a bad case of whooping cough to recover the joy of living. Another no longer responds to immaterial doses after a case of mumps.

Ever since Dr Voll's work these failures have ceased to be a mystery, at least for the few homoeopaths who are aware of energetic realities. The ohmmeter permits measurement of certain bioelectric variations that occur after childhood illness where the morbid explosion has not followed the strict natural model. But the machine detects only the major traces. Those that are more delicate, often more treacherous, escape the doctor completely if he has not been able to raise his consciousness to the energetic level of Life.

Of all the refined techniques that permit this delicate psychosensorial approach, radiesthesia is unquestionably the best. It combines speed and elegance, while not being restrictive for the patient. It demands, however, a certain aptitude in the practitioner, that can be learned only through suffering and a degree of sacrifice. When I finally abandoned the deceptive ease of Voll's method, I understood that no electronic technique could equal the qualities of human perception. And I discovered what no master had taught me – that all specific childhood illnesses can leave an etheric trace that is real and can be clearly identified. This is true even for common chicken-pox or a poor, insignificant case of German measles lasting only 3 days.

I therefore took the decision that had become self-evident: since the isopathic correction of significant shocks brought such a tremendous relief to the patients, why not erase the little shocks as well? And so I gave my patients (even the healthy ones) the respective nosodes of these illnesses that I had discovered through anamnesis or through the artifice of radiesthesia. Naturally this was done in strict respect of the inverse chronology required by my sequential logic.

The results were extraordinary. The simple fact of giving the German measles nosode at the right moment to an apparently healthy and perfectly balanced person can cause an enormous nose–throat elimination if childhood German measles have left a secret mark that is not accessible with Voll's method. Another example is the whooping cough nosode, which can make a healthy old man declared in perfect balance by the most sensitive ohmmeter cough beyond belief. All the nosodes given in this way to people who apparently had no need for them started a real process of toxic elimination. And at the end of this cleaning programme, all my patients, whether they had been chronically or only slightly ill, remarked that their general condition had been vastly improved once the inevitable preliminary worsening had passed. This is when I realized that the theory of barriers according to Voll and the others was only a rough approximation of morbid realities, and I distanced myself definitively from it at this time.

Beginning in 1975, I replaced this simplistic notion with the more critical vision of a successive layered stickiness that prevents the free flow of vital energy. I understood that each specific event adds its own undesired energy to the harmonious cluster of our complex spatiotemporal flux, deviating and restraining its serene flow. By 'specific event' I mean any extraneous wave whose characteristics of length and amplitude don't exactly correspond to those of the superior wave. It is obvious that a common throat or ear infection, or even bronchopneumonia, do not constitute in themselves this kind of breakdown in harmony. They are merely missed notes in the performance of a symphony, and are quickly forgiven. Only major events threaten the coherence of the whole, and it is clearly childhood illnesses that present the greatest risk of confusing the still unfamiliar partition of the early years of life. It is prudent to dig them out and erase their discordant traces as quickly as possible. A proper treatment must erase them all.

To help you better understand the serious damage sometimes caused, I will now change perspective. I won't continue to subject you to fastidious lists of eloquent clinical cases as proof of the opinions I am expressing. Instead I will simply present the method of treatment that I recommend when parents announce one of these illnesses to me by phone. You will immediately grasp the obvious superiority of Real Medicine, and the very real dangers to which an ordinary treatment exposes these little patients.

Smallpox and BCG vaccinations have already been the targets of my criticism. The two new subjects that concern me are scarlet fever and measles.

SCARLET FEVER

When the paediatrician suspects a case of scarlet fever in one of his young patients, there is an immediate generalized alarm, not to say panic. Complete quarantine, throat smears for the whole family, anxious anticipation of the verdict and finally an absolute and unquestionable decision: powerful antibiotics for all germ-carriers and anti-inflammatories for the feverish victim. You will shortly discover the consequences of all this activity.

When I learn of a similar misfortune with one of my patients the scenario at the beginning is the same, but minus the fear. As soon as we get into the counter-attack everything changes. First of all there is a distinction: if the child has only recently been introduced to homoeopathy (or put more colourfully, if he is not yet in orbit), I let his usual paediatrician take care of him and I repair the inevitable damage afterwards. But if the child has already been thoroughly 'purged' by my treatment and has a good energetic balance, I assume control of the operations.

First of all, what is scarlet fever? It is the frightening clinical picture presented by a child's organism when its vital energy has been surprised by a particularly aggressive variety of a common streptococcus that has been living with us since the beginning of time. It is the ferocious war that destroys a civilization when the capital's defences have been penetrated by a Trojan horse. A handful of Greek warriors conquers the sleeping troops, and erases with blood any memory of prior neighbourly relations.

How can this drama be prevented? How can the defences be organized? There is a simple solution: alert the guards in time and mobilize the troops before it is too late. It is a question requiring precise and speedy intelligence gathering and its rapid transmission. This information must reach the commanding officer immediately. The allopathic doctor feels comfortable because he has spotted the enemy quickly and has a powerful weapon to use against the aggressor: antibiotics. He is dramatically wrong. This aid always reaches the besieged citadel too late because it is not the doctor who needs the information, but King Priam who is asleep in his secret chamber and is the only one able to order a general mobilization. A homoeopath is able to wake him up, with great suddenness. No medication can transmit information as quickly as the immaterial dose, not even cortisone. The impact of a high potency is shattering and it has the essential quality required: precision.

A strong case of scarlet fever always presents a fairly spectacular picture: high fever, sudden apparition, agitation, scarlet colouring, etc. In Hahnemann's portrait gallery, its immaterial double is quickly found: Belladonna. An immediate dose of this remedy in a high potency transmits a precise image of the adversary to all concerned.

Now let us look at what happens afterwards. As soon as the pills carrying the Belladonna energy melt on the tongue, a coded message is instantly carried as a spatiotemporal quantum along the olfactory and gustatory nerves to the brain. There it enters the holiest of holies, the secret headquarters of the general. This message instantaneously describes and even exaggerates the horrors of the scarlet war. With Belladonna I have more or less painted the devil on the wall. The general's reaction? There is a moment of anxiety and then war is declared. No one is overlooked. The army, police, militias and even isolated snipers are immediately thrown into battle, and what a battle it is! A real massacre! No germ in the world can resist such a war-like fever. A battalion of commandos can't survive an assault from the entire armed forces.

Total victory is guaranteed with this single preliminary measure. All the defensive actions follow the master plan coded by Belladonna. The fever might remain high for a few days: all the better! It will make the germs' survival that much harder since they don't stand up very well to heat. (In giving Belladonna I always specify that it is not to bring down the fever, but to channel the defensive energies in the right direction.) The child is depressed and excited at the same time. He must stay in bed. If he is thirsty he can drink. If he is not hungry, all the better! His vital energy has more important things to do. The feasting Trojans were not a lot of help in defending their city from attack. The throat inflammation is extreme, the glands are swollen, and the skin becomes intensely red and finally peels.

I usually complement the activity of this first remedy with Mercurius solubilis if the swollen throat is serious, give Rhus toxicodendron if the itching is too uncomfortable and always prescribe copper, the important biological catalyst that brings its precious help in an immunological counter-attack. If the constitution is really too weak, I reinforce everything with serocytol therapy. I use these arms because they are available in all nearby pharmacies, but there are of course many other natural means available to reinforce homoeopathy. One only needs to ask the advice of a competent pharmacist not entirely dependent on the chemical industry for his survival.

With this kind of treatment scarlet fever doesn't leave too unpleasant a memory behind. It 'comes out' completely through the skin in perfect respect of Hering's Law. Recovery is thus ensured and the precious nerve, heart and kidney cells are unaffected. Later complications need not be feared. The child recovers his complete vitality a week after this lightning war and sometimes even after a few days, to the great surprise of all concerned.

Naturally this outstanding success can occur only if the homoeopath has really done his job properly as a family doctor. If the child's vital energy has been stuck for a long time in a heavy history of accumulated imbalances, there will not be the possibility of shaking it up with these subtle remedies; it will not be able to react. The doctor will have to resort to antibiotics even if he believes himself to be a homoeopathic virtuoso. (This type of failure, which is fairly frequent and often pointed to by allopaths, does not prove the inefficacy of our doses, but merely the incompetence of the practitioner who has failed to correct the patient's energetic balances in a timely manner.)

Another absolute requirement for success is the timeliness of the homoeopathic riposte. If the dose of Belladonna is given too late, the result isn't so good because the attackers have already overcome the defence. This is why I give all the families who have entrusted me with their care a dose of Belladonna XMK in reserve, and I recommend that they purchase an emergency kit of homoeopathic remedies once the sequential treatment is well advanced.

This is therefore the treatment that I give to my little patients. Fortunately there are very few who catch this illness, since children with a good energetic balance resist the haemolytic streptococcus better than the others, and are often only passive carriers of the germs. But, as with those who are really ill, I also force these children to one final effort. Three weeks after the infection, I give the nosode Scarlatinum XMK, to erase for ever the distortion inflicted by this war on the vital energy's spatiotemporal transmissions. With this final and indispensable act I eliminate the remaining risk of complications or relapse, since the enemy is now known, identified at general headquarters and no longer able to surprise the guards.

Now let us take a look at the 'official' treatment. Since Alexander Fleming it can be summarized in one word: penicillin.

Antibiotic therapy has ushered medicine into a new era. Penicillin and its derivatives have completely conquered the bacterial illnesses of childhood, and it cannot be denied that the mortality rate from scarlet fever has dropped in a spectacular way since use of these drugs has become universal. The related and much feared side-effects are now also a thing of the past.

Alas, however, this great triumph is only an illusion! If over-vaccination is the major imposture of our medical dogma, then systematic antibiotic therapy is its greatest mistake. Its triumphant dissemination is based on an enormous misunderstanding, which will in its turn be severely judged by future generations. The presentation here of a few basic truths, not very well known by either doctors or public, may well help clarify ideas entangled in polemical discussions.

Let us face reality. Before Fleming, millions of human beings caught scarlet fever without lasting damage, and thousands died of it. Why this cruel distinction? Because the first group had the benefit of a good energetic balance at the time of their infection, while the others had lost it earlier. This is obvious. With antibiotics these unfortunate people now have the support of heavy artillery that has been brought in to kill the attackers. At least that is what the doctors think.

In reality, antibiotic treatment functions less owing to its direct action against germs (which it kills or prevents from spreading) than by the shock it gives the defence systems (somewhat like the neuroendocrine impulse associated with stress), providing welcome encouragement in the effort to overcome the many unruly and resistant germs. When vital energy is seriously destabilized, the antibiotic shock always has some effect. This was well known to Allied pilots during the World War II who injected themselves with precious penicillin in order to 'keep going' after the serious shock of an otherwise straightforward and clean wound!

This very real shock is beneficial if it is powerful and brief. This is why it can completely stop the beginning of a flu even though this infection is not caused by bacteria but by viruses, which are perfectly insensitive to penicillin! But this rapid advantage is always paid at too high a price. The substance is toxic for all living germs, good and bad. When one realizes that our entire nutritional system depends on the enormous work of billions of intestinal bacteria, one can also have enough intelligence to avoid disturbing this wonderful ecosystem with killer molecules. There has never been medication that was so well deserving of its name. *Anti* and *bios* come from Greek: 'Beware! You are acting *against life.*'

I fully recognize and accept that this powerful treatment conquered infectious illnesses. It is the last resort that our deplorable materialist medicine deserved. As long as it goes on denying vital energy, it is unable to heal by intelligent regulation of the disturbed balance. It succeeds despite itself, almost against its own wishes, by counting on the secondary and flashy drug effects which it mistakenly takes for primary effects. But this misunderstanding can't last. Germs themselves are living organisms and know how to adapt to their environment. They are increasingly able to escape antibiotics and take new forms that are completely insensitive to chemotherapy. When all material arms have been rendered inoperative, the half-doctors will finally be forced to learn the other half of our art.

But let us go back to scarlet fever. The antibiotic treatment rapidly destroys the major part of the battalion of aggressive streptococci; the throat inflammation diminishes and the fever drops immediately. The invaders haven't had time to pour their terrible toxins into the bloodstream. The vital organs have been spared and the danger has been avoided. The child recovers quickly, at least in appearance, and goes back to school.

This is the description of the ideal and extremely rare case. Most of the time things don't quite happen this way. Antibiotic treatment always deeply disturbs the subtle balance of the various germ populations of the intestinal tract. When the harmony of coexistence is unstable any minor mishap can cause a catastrophe, and chemical bombardment is not just a minor mishap. Even when it is accompanied by the ingestion of yeasts to help repair the damage, it still can't help but contribute to the schisms that indirectly eat away at the cohesiveness of an intestinal ecosystem already under enough duress in this century of universal agroalimentary chemical pollution.

Most of the time the child is therefore very tired after this assisted battle. Sometimes he even becomes weaker, the convalescence prolongs itself and interest in work and play disappears. I have often seen these intense states of fatigue go on for 2, 4 and even 6 months following a case of scarlet fever that has been 'cut-off' with penicillin. What has happened?

The antibiotic can't kill all the pathogenic germs. Since it abruptly stops the fever through its direct impact on the adrenal glands they can no longer protect against the sneaky proliferation of the germs that escape. If the child is robust his vital energy, though shaken by the antibiotic stress, will be able to control the situation after a more or less lengthy convalescence. The pathogenic germs will all be destroyed. But for a somewhat weaker child the chemical assistance will initially have helped restore the missing balance but will never be able to provide the additional energy necessary to take complete control over the clandestine germ colonies that have survived the massacre. These continue to undermine the body's delicate immunological surveillance systems with their toxic emissions.

Exhausted and depressed, these children are destined to a morose future of chronic rheumatism or cardiovascular disease. Remember Christophe's story. There will be increasing numbers of children overwhelmed by the commonplace invaders of childhood. Given one or two more generations subjected to the French malaise, to overvaccination and intensive chemotherapy, and the entire world will be colonized by these arrogant germs. One doesn't have to search further for an explanation to the continuous and widespread increase of these illnesses so characteristic of the general morbidity of the close of this 20th century.

You think that I'm exaggerating again? My concepts are too different from those of the faculty to be credible? Then explain to me why there are never any complications interfering with my little patients' recoveries, even with children who are so fragile that they can no longer stand any type of iatrogenic shock. I invite my learned colleagues to explain why I often start off a tremendous scarlet fever with temperature, shivers, swollen throat and even contagion when I give the Scarlatinum nosode to one of their ex-patients who had been 'cured' with antibiotics 1 or even 20 years earlier. Why are there so many relapses of scarlet fever? Today two or three relapses are no longer uncommon if the child is treated according to dogma. How do you explain, professors, that after taking my nosode (a placebo according to you), an old patient's skin can become intensely red and peel abundantly ... 40 years after the first infection? But then you will only understand the nature of this observation (extremely commonplace in isotherapy) the day you are able to look in the impartial mirror of reality.

I must further specify something concerning this very peculiar illness. When I find it mentioned in the anamnesis of patients who have come to see me for entirely different reasons, I obviously include the Scarlatinum nosode in its appropriate place in my isotherapeutic sequence. But this corrective measure is sometimes inadequate. Since this illness has invariably been treated by the imperious treatment of the preceding colleague I must also add another isotherapeutic to my treatment, the simile of the penicillin that often significantly alters the shape of scarlet fever's wave. The simple fact of this reversed antibiotic shock is then often enough to unleash the virulence of the scarlet distortion that was only lightly shackled by the chemical artifice.

A last example will help you to understand this commonplace reality of my daily practice better than any theoretical explanation. On 9 December 1983 I saw Nathalie T, a lovely little girl aged 10 years who had been suffering since spring from pruritis of the vulva that was truly unbearable. Various examinations had found nothing in particular. The paediatrician had thought of worms and ordered a vermifuge, but with no success. The anamnesis revealed a common sequence of natural and iatrogenic destabilizing shocks and I began the sequential treatment: Varicellinum for the chicken-pox of December 1978, then Parotidinum in January 1984 for the mumps of September 1978, the nosode of rabies in February for a vaccine taken in 1977, then Rubeolinum for the German measles of 1976 and finally in May, Morbillinum for the measles at age 3. On 26 June I gave her Penicillinum to erase the shock of the 1975 scarlet fever treatment ... and in so doing poked a stick right into the middle of the hornet's nest. The itching became burning, urination was painful, the vulva turned bright red, the labia were badly ulcerated. The situation was critical. Why? Because I had gone back through time to the key moment, the scarlet fever at age 2 that had been 'cut' too quickly by the doctrinaire haste of her paediatrician. On 9 July I finally gave the Scarlatinum nosode in XMK. It was like a magic wand!

Immediately after taking the immaterial remedy the child complained about her throat, which became red, the itching reached a peak, a genital discharge took place, the vulva peeled, as did the feet and even the buttocks! This uncomfortable aggravation lasted 48 hours, then at the beginning of the 3rd day all the symptoms definitively disappeared. Nathalie recovered the boundless energy that her parents remembered. She was cured. I will let you imagine how her life would have been if the proper isotherapy had not re-established her energetic balance. It most certainly would have been demolished between dermatologists, urologists, gynaecologists and finally psychiatrists, with sterility a real possibility and morosity a certainty.

Examples like this of infant gynaecology are not rare. Every year I see at least one little girl afflicted with a suspicious discharge. Each time I find scarlet fever deeply buried under successive layers of spatiotemporal stickiness. I am certain that if the doctors took the time to look there are at least 20 or 30 cases like this every year in the city of Lausanne alone. The same quantity of 'inexplicable' chronic pyelonephritis would also be found, along with odd heart murmurs, painful swollen articulations, sudden obesity, incomprehensible diabetes and severe depressions. For such a small city, that adds up to a lot of people who are very young and very ill. If you multiply this number by the number of other towns, villages and cities, and you will have an idea of the millions of people who would be freed from their miseries by Real Medicine.

I will not say more here about scarlet fever. Each of these diagnoses could be illustrated with an evocative example, but I must save a little space to discuss another of my *bêtes noires*: measles. I can now be somewhat briefer since my reasoning and that of allopathic doctors can be superposed exactly as in the case of scarlet fever.

MEASLES

The agent responsible for measles is not a bacterium, but a virus. The paediatricians are therefore not able to deploy their full arsenal since, as everyone knows, viruses don't react to antibiotics. Only an ass would use these useless weapons (and yes, I've often seen it done). The others confine themselves to using anti-inflammatories to stop the beneficial fever, the glandular congestion sought by nature, and the pain.

For a real doctor, the treatment of measles is child's play and can be outlined by telephone if the diagnosis is certain. (The paediatrician can at least provide this service.) As with scarlet fever first give the dose of Belladonna XMK from your homoeopathic medicine chest. It is the ideal remedy at the beginning of measles. All by itself it will mobilize the defences in the right direction. The skin eruption can be significantly increased by this. All the better! There is never any reason to be afraid of cutaneous reactions: they are the best proof that Hering's Law has been respected.

If the child is congested and swollen, give Pulsatilla in small doses. If the eyes are intensely irritated, give Euphrasia. If swallowing is painful, add Mercurius solubilis and Phytolacca if the glands are really painful. That's all. With a child who is habitually in good health – ie energetically well balanced – measles that are treated this way are not the slightest problem. I have taken care of several hundred in this manner without recourse to even the slightest chemical molecule. All those children did very well. In fact mothers quickly become expert in using the small homoeopathic doses and regain the confidence in nature that their paediatricians had destroyed. The spectre of complications that these paediatricians brandish can only frighten people (unfortunately too numerous) not yet acquainted with Real Medicine.

Whether I am asked to help or not, the one urgent request that I have concerning any childhood illness is that I be advised of its occurrence. Remember, this type of illness is an important event. As with scarlet fever, I must give the Morbillinum nosode 21 days after the outbreak in order to erase for ever the astral distortion and prevent long-term complications and relapses. In fact it doesn't matter if I am advised later, since it is the initial 3-week period that counts. If the nosode is given too quickly the natural immunity from the illness would be compromised and might therefore not protect the child from a relapse.

MUMPS

For mumps, the scenario is identical – first Belladonna, to 'ripen' the infection, then often Ferrum phosphoricum to avoid hormonal complications. For this I also often give zinc–nickel–cobalt which is extremely efficient. Gelsemium is indispensable if there is a meningeal risk, and is always enough to avoid this problem. Hamamelis prevents swelling of the testicles or ovaries, which I take care of if necessary with serocytol therapy. Pulsatilla and Phytolacca are often useful and diminish congestion. If the swelling is enormous and the pain intense, I also give an anti-inflammatory, but not that of the chemists. There are three or four vegetal enzyme specialities available on the market, which are well tolerated and efficient. My preference is for Traumanase whose active principal is a pineapple extract.

That's it. Naturally, 3 weeks after the outbreak, the Parotidinum nosode must also be given. This is essential since without this corrective erasure the risk of endocrinological complications would be too great, particularly with carbonics of the Graphites type or with ultra sensitive phosphorics.

OTHER CHILDHOOD ILLNESSES

It remains for me to describe the minor illnesses: chicken-pox, whooping cough, German measles and, the last of the major childhood illnesses, diphtheria. This latter is no longer amongst us now that everyone has been vaccinated. It is therefore not the illness that I treat, but the energetic sequels left by the vaccine. The perfect treatment is the Diphtherinum nosode, prepared from a culture of the germs that cause the illness.

Chicken-pox is not very harmful even though it involves the mucous membranes and is quite spectacular. A few doses of Rhus toxicodendron are usually enough to 'ripen' it and reduce the itching (Mezereum is also very effective); three weeks later I give Varicellinum, of course.

Whooping cough is quite rare as we saw, and inoffensive if the child is energetically in balance. Small vegetal remedies like Drosera, Coccus cacti and Sambucus are enough to control the bothersome cough. Much more frequent is the iatrogenic case from overvaccination. The half-doctors try very hard to remove the symptoms, but to no avail. Only a real doctor can get to the bottom of the problem by giving the Pertussinum nosode.

As for German measles it is so insignificant for a child in good health that the parents usually forget even to mention it to me. Nevertheless this must be done as I won't have a clear conscience until the Rubeolinum nosode has been taken in the usual time-frame.

This concludes my review of childhood illnesses. I have presented them in decreasing order of importance. The other small childhood fevers have not been included since they do not leave an imprint.

All other infectious illnesses are treatable in the same manner. The much-feared viral hepatitis, salmonellosis and brucellosis are no longer terrible calamities, charged with uncontrollable consequences. The period of convalescence is considerably shortened to the great surprise of the non-believers who are devoted to materialist science. And as for infectious mononucleosis, or glandular fever, the 'student's illness' when I was young; it now strikes younger and younger children, sometimes causing leukaemia in children treated by allopathic doctors. When countered with our energetic arms, its simple treatment is transformed into an instructive and gratifying game.

I still routinely use chemical weapons in cases of toxoplasmosis, venereal disease, amoebiosis and parasitosis, but I carefully limit the damage through a vigorous homoeopathic scrubbing of the toxic residues that are left by these foreign molecules. And naturally I also periodically and willingly use penicillin – thank-you Sir Alexander Fleming! – when a patient's life seems to me to be in danger. This type of extreme emergency is very rare in my practice (once or twice a year), since like an imperial Chinese mandarin I pride myself on attending to the preservation of my patients' energetic balances. More frequently it is the general panic of the family or the aggressiveness of the patient that results in the prescription of other antibiotics that are not really necessary.

Finally, I admit that it is impossible to avoid totally the use of allopathic medicine during the first weeks of my new patient's initiation. This also holds true for the hundred or so patients who remain from my old internist's practice, and whom I was unable to adapt to the reactional mode of homoeopathy. They are usually older people whose illnesses have become chronic. The chemical remedies I prescribe for them each month would fit comfortably into a large suitcase. I would be incapable of putting together the same volume of chemicals in a year for the thousands of other people I heal with my sequential therapy!

This glaring, measurable disparity is the best image I can give of the materialistic grossness of ordinary treatments when compared with the subtle yet vivid immateriality of Real Medicine.

FIFTEEN

The major shocks

When doctors finally decide to free humanity from the immaterial after-effects of overvaccination and childhood illnesses, the deserted hospitals can be used for the homeless and other disinherited of the Earth. These after-effects that stay with us for an entire lifetime are by far the most important cause of the general energetic destabilization that is at the root of all illness. But they are not alone in diminishing our resistance. Other factors are of course at work too – important 'events' that leave their cruel, permanent and active traces in our different memory systems.

To awaken your interest in these, a brief overview was contained in Chapter 9, and I would now like to take you through some of my archives to illustrate certain of them with real-life examples. I feel compelled to point out at least the most common of these active troublemakers. Curiously, they are often the same that simple folk-wisdom points to in such phrases as: 'Nothing has been the same since my accident' or 'since my operation in 1981' or 'since I lost my wife'. Most doctors consider these precious revelations as idle talk and shrug their shoulders. The common sense of 'ordinary people' is closer to the truth than their learned devitalized reasoning. In the example that follows, the impact of the event is so clear that even my most obstinate colleagues would be unable to deny its importance.

On 6 April 1981, while travelling on vacation, Mlle Brigitte M, aged 21, was the victim of a bad traffic accident near Marseilles. She was taken to the hospital in a critical condition. The cranial shock was severe, and 5 weeks in intensive care had been unable to correct the altered consciousness. She was brought back to Switzerland and hospitalized at the major cantonal hospital in

Lausanne where she remained for many long, cruel weeks. At the time of her discharge the EEG was finally more or less normal, but her entire life had been turned upside down.

The neurological sequels of her long coma were not completely erased. Surgery had corrected the strabismus that had appeared following the accident, but the pupils were still unequal. Her character had changed and she had become aggressive, complaining of painful headaches and an inability to concentrate. She abandoned her studies. In addition, she was always cold, often constipated and gaining weight inexplicably.

I first saw her in November 1983, more than 2½ years after the drama. The neurological aftermaths were very visible and her grievances seemed to be fully justified. People close to her confirmed that life in her proximity had become intolerable ... and they expected me to perform a miracle.

It is not easy for a doctor to become involved in the destiny of a patient for whom medicine has declared that nothing can be done. But, faced with this type of situation every week, I do not give up hope. I now know that life has more than one trick up its sleeve.

The first assessment was not very encouraging. On the right-hand side the vital energy seemed to flow normally through the meridians, but since the patient was left-handed, it was by the left hand that I had to judge. And what I found confirmed the suspected energetic catastrophe. There was nothing at all! All the meridians were disconnected and the current of life no longer passed.

Like a policeman, I started my investigation. But not, like them, at the scene of the crime. For me the scope also had to include the highly destabilizing events that had occurred since the accident. Experience had taught me that, like the firemen's water after a fire, the doctors' 'vigorous' treatments could be at least as damaging as any accident. Once I had all the information I retained a few key suspects from among the many violent events that had marked those hours and days of anxiety. There were six: the shock of fear, the cranial shock doubled with the loss of consciousness, the operation associated with the ophthalmological operation, the cortisone, the X-rays, and the lack of adequate oxygen to the brain over a prolonged period.

Six corresponding immaterial entities had to be found that carried the same energetic charge programmed backwards. In order, they were Opium, Arnica and Natrum sulphuricum, Nux vomica, Cortisonum, X-ray and Ammonium carbonicum. It took me 5 months and six visits to pass this six-part message, and it was like the work of a watchmaker, requiring a great deal of patience and rigorous reasoning.

At the seventh visit on 30 April 1984, the miracle happened! The liberated vital energy flowed freely along the meridians and had recovered its balance. Three years after the accidental blockage the clock of higher space–time once again emitted its regulating ticking: Yin calling Yang and Yang leading Yin.

I had used only my ten fingers, my pendulum, six immaterial doses and zinc–nickel–cobalt. In addition, at the beginning of the treatment I had prescribed Jaunitine, a wonderful mix of selected herbs that I often use to ensure an adequate draining of the biliary system. That's all. I am not hiding anything. These modest means were enough to re-establish hope and change the course of destiny. This young woman recovered a good part of her intellectual abilities and, although the neurological sequels are not yet entirely erased, they no longer represent absolutely irreversible damage and are fading gradually from month to month.

This example was chosen to spare you five other stories. Each of the six events mentioned is in itself important and sufficient to destroy an entire life if the disturbance it creates permanently suffocates the vital energy. In this exceptional case, the young woman would never have recovered if I had left one of them out.

Luckily, every case of concussion or surgical operation does not have this destructive power. If the vital energy is powerful and well balanced, the traumatic event leaves merely a passing vestige and the individual retains it only as a vague memory. Nevertheless I ask all my patients to advise me of similar events within a reasonably short period (days or weeks) in order to avoid the possible severity of an enduring trace. I then send them a repairing homoeopathic dose. With events that can be planned, such as an imminent operation, I always give my patients a combined dose of Arnica and Nux vomica in 200K to take just before the intervention, and the same mixture in MK to take as soon as they wake up. Without exception they have told me that they had never felt as well in waking up after an operation.

Material shocks are a tangible and painful reality. However, there is another category of traumatism that does even more harm, even though it leaves no visible wounds. I refer here to the terrible trials that life can put before us, the cruel losses from which one never really recovers. One popular song says that they 'bruise the soul'. Doctors should be able to diagnose these as well, and in addition should be able to heal them. Instead drugs are added to the sadness, when the wounds of the soul merely ask to be relieved.

What is a memory? It is merely the trace of an important event that is inscribed on a space–time network. To remove this trace the same event has to be imprinted on the other side of the cloth. To exorcize a pain that is still vivid one must have the courage to live through it again backwards in time. Confessors, psychotherapists and charitable friends devote themselves to this task but nothing can replace the unequalled efficiency of a correctly chosen and dynamized homoeopathic dose. Of all the medication invented by humanity it is the only one to have this wonderful power of going back through time.

On 6 October 1978 I had an emergency visit from Mme X, treated since 1962 by a reputed homoeopath who had been forced to reduce his activities considerably. I was therefore asked to take over her care with an additional request that I be particularly careful in dosing my remedies since she was apparently ultrasensitive to homoeopathy and couldn't stand doses above 200K. Intrigued by this warning I examined the medical file and was quite amazed to see that the previous doctor had indeed never dared go beyond 200K and had spent the prior 16 years doing nothing but fortify her fragile constitution with alternate doses of Silicea, Petroleum, and Graphites at 30K. He nevertheless was periodically brave enough to prescribe enormous doses of Pulsatilla, a remedy that is generally well supported by the most delicate constitutions. (Homoeopathic preparations of plant origin are very gentle and harmonize vital energy without the roughness of those of animal origin or the sharpness of those from the mineral order.) I found only one isopathic intervention in the entire file, and it had certainly been dictated by the ohmmeter: the erasure of a childhood whooping cough. There was no mention, let alone correction, of any of the important events that had marked this woman's life.

The homoeopath had been guided through the years by the clinical symptoms and by Voll's technique. He had done reasonably well in maintaining a precarious balance by giving doses for the constitution (more about this in Part III), but had been unable in 16 years to prevent his patient from sinking imperceptibly into a deeply imbalanced energetic situation which was manifesting itself in the form of a crisis.

Why this failure? Because the doctor, unaware of the spatiotemporal continuity of vital energy, had without knowing it violated the fundamental law of the art of healing, which must be rigorously respected by all homoeopaths: Hering's Law, which must be respected to the letter.

The crisis that had provoked this urgent request for a first consultation turned out to be a commonplace migraine of cervical origin accompanied by disagreeable nausea and dizziness. It was simply the sign of the progressive establishment of arthrosis that neither the doctor nor his patient had been able to stop. This first alert was brought under control by a wonderful old bone-setter from our neighbouring Gruyère, Mme Rose Scherly who has since passed away. Things took a less celestial turn when the treatment continued in my office. The preliminary investigations were difficult since my patient wasn't able to reply with the precision I wanted and continuously repeated herself, advancing insignificant details and forgetting important ones. Her memory seemed to be confused and her state of nervous fatigue was painful to observe. Her nights were filled with dreadful nightmares and her condition was always at its worst on waking up in the morning. She was exhausted, depressed and suffering from extreme anxiety. What a wonderful advertisement for homoeopathy!

You've already guessed the reason for this terrible waste: the constant imbalance of vital energy. One of Voll's followers would certainly speak here of blockage and find a plausible guilty party with the ohmmeter, depending on his inspiration. I refrain from Voll's temptation and prefer to use my own method of chronological detection, which is simultaneously more intuitive and more rigorous. The first outstanding event in this backwards countdown was a primary tubercular infection in my patient that had occurred rather late in life following two very painful periods of mourning. I immediately understood why she had so often been considered 'Pulsatilla' since this remedy indicates a tubercular constitution. Her doctor had in fact prescribed a homoeopathic dose of tuberculin in 1973 in the hope of correcting this weakness. Unfortunately he made a terrible mistake in prescribing an inappropriate version of the remedy. The bovine tuberculin that he administered, no doubt based on certain ohmmetric readings, had merely exacerbated a hereditary constitution that shouldn't have been disturbed before it was time. The patient became even more Pulsatilla than before and was precipitated into 5 years of increasing imbalance.

The remedy for primary tubercular infection that I have most frequently identified in my investigations is called Tuberculinum humanum. After verification with radiesthesia I gave Mme X this first correction to her balance in a very high potency. Given correctly, at the right time and in respect of the Law, there can be no intolerance.

I saw the patient again in March 1979. She was transformed. Her energetic balance was still very precarious, but the general picture was no longer Pulsatilla. I was now looking at a living portrait of Ignatia. Open a book with the homoeopathic Materia Medica and read: Ignatia is the remedy of changing moods, melancholia and neurasthenia causing unjustified swings from laughter to tears, sighs to palpitations. All manuals propose this remedy in cases of emotional trouble following a death. It is almost the specific antidote of cruel sorrow. The event immediately preceding – and unquestionably the cause of – my patient's primary tubercular infection, was the loss of her dearly loved parents. She collapsed in tears at the mere mention of this painful event even though many years had since passed. I immediately understood that the immaterial trace was very much alive and significantly interfering with the guiding transmissions of higher energy.

I applied the simple treatment on the spot: Ignatia in a very high potency to go back through time with the required strength and speed. In so doing I removed the grain of sand that was preventing the harmonious unfolding of life. Mme X has since regained a perfect energetic balance and willingly underwent my complementary sequential treatment. She withstood without difficulty the high potencies administered between 1980 and 1983. They cleared her past of all its iatrogenic and natural barriers and with her regained energy she was able to deal courageously with a difficult life.

This example shows the healing effect of a homoeopathic dose that is directed solely to the psyche. It is totally efficient when the destabilizing event has only affected the mental sphere. But there is another type of psychological shock, exclusively feminine, that is coupled with an additional physically painful and profoundly destabilizing wound. Since this situation is far more common than people think, I will give a brief example reinforced in its spectacular aspects by the usually incurable nature of the problem.

Mme Y came to see me in 1973 following a suggestion from an ENT surgeon friend. He had been as unsuccessful as his predecessors in removing the terrible symptoms that cause so many suicides. The young woman had been suffering from a terrible trigeminal neuralgia for the past 6 years. All the classical treatments had been tried in vain. Nothing from the common anti-inflammatories of the internist to the very sophisticated drugs of the neurologist and the meticulous intervention of a neurosurgeon had worked. Acupuncture and diverse manipulations of the cervical column had been a disappointment. The young woman was condemned to daily doses of tranquillizers and had begun to wonder whether life was really worth living.

At the time I was still only a half-doctor, but had already acquired a certain reputation for my use of 'gentle' techniques. I tried to diminish the intense pain with prolonged serocytol therapy combined with biological catalysis. The first results were encouraging and 1974 brought some hope. But by 1976 the pain was back even stronger than before and my patient returned for more help.

Having by this time completed the other half of my medical knowledge I was better armed to find an efficient parry. An enormous energetic imbalance was immediately apparent to the doctor that I had become. The vital energy no longer flowed along the main meridian. What was causing this total breakdown? With such a young and apparently robust patient it couldn't be a minor incident. I minutely re-examined the anamnesis in the new light of Real Medicine and ran right into the most recent event of importance that had taken place several years before the apparition of the neuralgia. The young woman confided to me in secret that she had interrupted an undesired pregnancy shortly before her marriage and retained a very vivid sense of guilt concerning this act. From my readings of the homoeopathic Materia Medica I remembered under China (quinquina) the following: 'corrects the effects of a large haemorrhage, an abortion or any important loss of organic matter'.

I immediately gave my tormented patient a high potency of this remedy ... and a miracle occurred. At the next visit she announced the disappearance of her ailment and told me that all her neuroleptic drugs had been thrown in the rubbish bin. Her recovery appears to be definitive since I have seen her every year since and have never had to deal with a relapse.

Naturally I can already hear behind my back the laughing chorus of those partisans of the placebo theory. It wasn't my medication that worked, but the catharsis of confession symbolized by little white purifying pills, etc ... But this time the laughter is really a little too much to bear. Gentlemen, here is the return thrust. My next little story should put the debate at its proper level: the austere arena of complete objectivity. The pedantic will not be able to find any psychological or pseudoscientific escape. There are no tricks and no speeches, only facts. Here they are.

One morning in 1977 as I went into the kitchen for breakfast I was surprised at not hearing the usual joyous whistles of greeting from Caprice, my daughter's guinea pig. Intrigued, I looked into the cage and found a very disconcerting picture. The little animal was lying on its side, inert in the middle of a brown and nauseous pool that had emptied from its intestines. With its glazed eyes, dull fur and the anus still completely open the animal seemed to be dead. In any case Caprice was clearly dying from the extreme dehydration caused by a severe diarrhoea. After 4 years with the little beast as our household mascot, I admit that I viewed this perspective with some dismay.

What to do? What can veterinary medicine do in such a situation? Suddenly the sentence I mentioned earlier came to my mind: 'any important loss of organic matter'. I rushed to my emergency medical kit which contained some China in 5C and clumsily stuck a few pills into the poor dry mouth of our pet before leaving for work. You can imagine my relief at lunchtime when I returned home and didn't find the animal dead. It was standing up on all four feet without moving, but the eyes and fur definitely looked a little more alive. My children had stopped crying and some hope had returned. I gave the animal a second stronger dose of the remedy in 200K. The end of the drama was near. By evening my household had recovered its good spirits. Caprice welcomed me home to dinner with her usual energy and the happy whistles that indicated a complete recovery. The dreadful and nauseous agony was a thing of the past and our pet was never again ill. She lived another 4 years, to the venerable age of 8, which is apparently quite honourable for members of this furry animal family.

The local university's pharmacology professor, who willingly appears in radio and television interviews to ridicule our art, will certainly be able to demonstrate to you that Caprice wholeheartedly believed in homoeopathy and thus allowed the placebo to work so effectively. Dear reader, I leave you to judge for yourself.

SIXTEEN

'Incurable' illnesses

The diversity of cases mentioned in this book may come as a surprise and give the impression that homoeopathy is able to heal all illnesses with equal ease. May the impression remain! It is my intention to bring about a change of heart on this score, as alas there is little doubt that an uninformed public considers homoeopathy capable of curing only trifling, unimportant illnesses. For many patients the reassuring armoury of the chemical industry seems essential when a situation is serious or critical.

With my examples I didn't necessarily want to demonstrate the superiority of one system over another, but rather that the essential aspect of the art of healing is, and always will be, the untiring search for energetic balance. It is solely the disharmony of vital energy that causes illness, benign or serious. I merely identified the most frequent causes of disturbance to this harmony.

It then becomes evident that the correct recognition of accumulated causes will allow a doctor to heal all illnesses, provided he has the means available to neutralize their effects. As we have seen, the iso- or homoeopathic remedy is the ideal weapon. However it isn't only the quality of the weapons used in a war that is essential, it is also critical to know when to intervene.

Our old friend time is constantly everywhere! It is the pivotal point of the present book, the secret spring of sequential therapy. Please forgive this brief passage explaining yet another imperative requirement of Real Medicine.

For the doctor, 'knowing when to intervene' means acting before the higher spatiotemporal continuum has completely lost control of the lower continuum. This is important because unfortunately the delicate space–time bridge joining these two limits can be trampled to such a point that it breaks. Professor Kozyrev's elastics also end up breaking beyond a certain point of tension. In life the breaking point has two aspects. When the spatial element goes first, the problem is surgical and an emergency. If the strain is essentially temporal, the problem is medical and chronic. In this case the breaking point is not as easily reached, leaving the doctor time to correct the distortion with his energetic treatment. As long as this breaking point is not reached, the illness remains functional and the corrective modalities are termed reactional. Recovery is both possible and enduring.

However if the treatment is started too late, beyond the infamous point, response to the healing impulse can only be passive and non-effective. The illness loses its functional characteristics and becomes lesional, requiring surgery or palliative medicine.

If you have grasped this, you now know why nothing seems impossible to a doctor who knows when to intervene. Since with sequential isotherapy he has a technique at hand that permits it, why should he deprive himself the pleasure of treating all kinds of sickness?

I want to share this joy with you through a final series of examples from my practice. The apparent disorder of this presentation is intentional. By contrast with the disparity of these diagnoses, I hope to reveal the constant superiority of Real Medicine.

Case 1.

In 1976 I saw André W, born in 1937, who had come to me with painful arthritis in his left big toe that, along with a lumbago, had appeared suddenly after he had been in a draught. We were both equally surprised by the lab tests. This was far more serious than an ordinary case of gout, since the analysis revealed traces of rheumatoid polyarthritis. This diagnosis threw a new light on the slight rheumatic problems elicited in the anamnesis that had been insufficient to convince the patient to see a doctor sooner. Now the situation was serious and energetic intervention necessary. When I was a young doctor this illness was called chronic progressive polyarthritis, a name that didn't hypocritically hide its doubly perverse nature. It warned the victim that it was in place for life and would worsen over time. This is unfortunately true if the patient puts himself in the hands of a 'specialist'. The affliction is in fact the perfect example of a 'sinecure' disorder, one that guarantees a comfortable lifelong income to rheumatologists and ends up making the surgeons wealthy as well.

At the time I didn't have a lot of experience with the therapeutic system that I had invented, and so I didn't dare assert to my patient that I would cure him. But his case seemed favourable, since no half-doctors had muddied the tracks ahead of me. André W gave me his full confidence, and we set out on an adventure that was to last 4 years and was full of ups and downs as painful as they were unexpected. First, all chemicals were put aside in favour of my usual weapons: nosodes, catalysts and vegetal buds.

I will skip the technical details of my interventions, which included the full range of all the anti-iatrogenic (forgive the expression) nosodes, the major draining remedies and all the isopathics of children's diseases. The high point of the treatment was reached as we negotiated the tightrope of the measles–scarlet fever duo. It was a real acrobatics without a net! In every case of polyarthritis that I have subsequently cured I have had to untangle the invisible and intricate sequels of these two diseases.

My patient passed through the tortures of some very spectacular aggravations: elbows, knees, fingers, jawbones and all the joints were a cruel source of suffering. One evening I even found him lying on his living room couch as the pain of moving had been too great for him to go to bed. But he held on, and V-Day ultimately arrived. Since March 1980 the battle has been won and his joints no longer refuse to give service.

In July 1982 there was a slight relapse of the illness in another form when it attacked the left eye. The ophthalmological clinic diagnosed an anterior uveitis and prescribed classic collyres (eye lotions), which the patient used for a few days. The recovery was very rapid, then was followed by a brief relapse in December. Rather than return to the oculist, the patient came to see me immediately. I gave him Mezereum 30 and 200K (this remedy works extremely well for inflammations of the left eye), and a day later the uveitis had disappeared. I am aware that the illness can reappear, but now we are solidly prepared for it. Since 1980 I have been fortifying the patient's constitution, and today he is considerably stronger than in 1976, with greater reactional capabilities. What is the reason for this victory? We succeeded because the patient came to see me before that infamous breaking point, and I was able to start the treatment in time.

Case 2.

On 18 January 1984 I received a visit from a little 6½-year-old girl named Stephanie P who suffered from mucoviscidosis. This diagnosis had been made at the paediatric clinic of the University of Geneva in 1980 and cannot be questioned. For the last 3 years the little patient had shown all the sad signs of this terrible affliction of genetic origin that thickens the pancreatic and bronchial secretions and leads to a progressive respiratory and digestive infirmity. This is true provided that knowledgeable technical medicine has been at work! Real Medicine can do better as you will see.

Before getting down to the genetic code, my first corrective interventions had to mend the distortions that had been directly inflicted on the child's life. This was quickly done. In the anamnesis I found only the inevitable, lamentable iatrogenic shocks: DTPP, DTPP, antibiotics, DTPP, antibiotics, DTPP, combined measles, mumps and German measles and finally a BCG vaccine. I started the treatment on the spot. It took all of February and March to erase the BCG shock. The manganese-copper catalyst helped to get through the first difficult phase and slightly diminished the stomach pains. At the beginning of April I drained the residual antibiotics and around mid-April removed the perverse waves of three artificial illnesses that struck at the wrong time with the measles–mumps–German measles vaccine. It then took me all of June to destroy the astral shell of the multiple DTPPs.

At the end of June I saw Stephanie again, and she had already changed. She was hungry and eating well while respecting her diet. Her meridians were perfectly balanced and she hadn't been ill since January. But there was still a significant facial asymmetry, with the left eye less open than the right. I prescribed an osteopathic correction and finally attacked the regulation of the genetic code.

Sulphur in 30 and 200K on 12 and 13 July opened fire. Then on 1 August I gave three doses of a remedy that I have invented and that is destined to model analogically the energetic structure of our genetic patrimony. I saw the little girl again on 19 September and she was transformed. Everyone around her said that it was like having another child come to life under their very eyes. There is already talk of expanding her diet, after a successful test with sausage. Just think about it for a moment. This was the first time that she had ever been able to taste such a food. Normally a deviation like this from her diet would have resulted in violent stomach pains. All hopes therefore suddenly seemed possible.

This first success was reinforced by the remarkable work of the osteopath. After a single session of cranial osteopathy the facial asymmetry had disappeared and the eyes had returned to their correct place. Such a concordance of positive achievements and such a synergy of corrective acts allowed one to imagine a favourable evolution, and who knows, a possible definitive stabilization. What is remarkable in this case are the rapid gains achieved through the anti-iatrogenic sequence and beginnings of the genetic treatment. University clinics don't manage a quarter of this in so short a time. The patients are hospitalized at enormous expense in specialized services and are studied by the professor, assistant professor and assistants, but the mucoviscidosis refuses to give up its secrets. For Stephanie, the real treatment started in September. I gave her the first important doses of Psorinum, the greatest of all the remedies inspired by Hahnemann and the most powerful of the genetic markers. With this first shock I decisively oriented the slow regulatory process in the way described in Part III of this book, and which has so often brought me an unhoped-for cure after 1, 2 or 3 years of sustained patience.

Case 3.

Here is another short story illustrating a distressing situation that has now become common in an internist's practice. On 7

November 1983 I saw a 39-year-old businessman named Philippe L who had been suffering from so-called 'essential' hypertension for 14 years. An illness receives this empty label when allopathic doctors have used up all the diagnostic resources of their art and have failed in the search for causes. For Philippe L, all the tests came up negative, and it hadn't been easy to find a palliative remedy. Finally, after a few years of chemical testing, the therapeutic choice fell upon a fashionable mixture of pills and the patient was condemned to taking them every day for the rest of his life.

Our patient, however, had a somewhat impatient character, and wasn't stupid. He was a rebel at heart and chose to abandon the treatments of the faculty. His story seemed very commonplace at the outset, like all anamneses. All destabilizing sequences resemble each other and yet each one is different. I started my corrective work right away. First Arnica for a recent shock, then Natrum sulphuricum for an older one, then Cortisonum in mid December for a stupid prior treatment of a false rheumatism. I saw the patient again in April. His blood pressure was normal at 11/9 and the tubes of pills had been thrown away since November. My treatment isn't finished yet, and I am continuing the sequential clean-up that will end sometime next year. But the blood pressure has never gone back up ... what a splendid example of 'essential' hypertension!

Case 4.

The first three illnesses mentioned above, reputed to be incurable by materialist medicine, affect tens of thousands of victims in the major countries of the West. The fourth illness I will mention affects several million.

Christiane V consulted me in March 1982 for buccal and genital herpes that had been tormenting her for 5 years. One hears a lot nowadays about this illness given that over the last few years it has spread increasingly quickly over the whole planet. It is caused by a virus from the large family of herpetic infections that includes chicken-pox, shingles, smallpox and vaccinia (cowpox). Allopathy doesn't have much to propose against this modern scourge. Viruses are resistant to antibiotics and are often stimulated by anti inflammatory drugs. What to do? The only attitude currently proposed, and which is commercialized for millions of dollars, is to ape homoeopathy: herpes is treated with a vaccine. But since it is nothing but an imitation, it can only bring relief, but never really cure. Only the homoeopathic potency is capable of elevating the vaccination to the superior energetic level where the harmony of our lives is ordered.

Christiane V had therefore not been cured. The vaccine had somewhat diminished the virulence of the symptoms, but had not been able to prevent numerous relapses. The anamnesis of the patient gave me a precise chronology of all the destabilizing events in her life and I began treatment immediately. Following the first four sequential shocks, the herpes was revived. In August 1982 I gave the fifth shock, the poliomyelitis nosode (Salk). The herpetic reaction was initially violent and then diminished. The sixth, seventh and eighth shocks passed unnoticed (Parotidinum, Tuberculinum humanum, Morbillinum), but the herpes had almost disappeared by the next visit on 1 February. Three events remained to be neutralized: Chicken-pox, the DiTePer and the vaccine. I feared a violent relapse since I was about to reactivate two viral cousins, but no eruption was awakened. At the September 1983 visit, the illness had disappeared. I continued with the regulation of the genetic code following my usual method, and completed my work in June 1984. In March, after taking one of my little packages of pills, the patient had noticed the appearance of a few small spots that quickly vanished. The herpes has never again appeared.

Case 5.

Far more serious is lupus erythematosus disseminatus. This illness, fortunately very rare, poses a difficult problem for scientific researchers who hesitate in attributing it to a viral agent (viral infection of the C type transmitted endogenetically since the beginning of time). Whatever the primary cause may be, its immunologically autodestructive apparitions progressively attack all the tissues and organs of its victims.

I can't help but think of the sad future that awaited Florian M, a young entrepreneur of 35 who sat before me one April morning in 1980. His lupus had first appeared at age 24 and was recognized fairly rapidly. The ridiculous treatment of the allopaths had been unable to prevent the slow worsening of the ailment. One by one the skin, kidneys and other organs had been affected. The skin became red and swollen and anti-inflammatories were applied. The joints were inflamed and bruised and the same reasoning was followed. The swelling reached the kidneys, eyes, and meninges. His blood was profoundly modified, its rate of sedimentation enough to make one dizzy. A last recourse to the ultimate anti-inflammatory weapon was decided: cortisone – the summum of 'medical' art.

The patient put up with this treatment for 6 months, during which time the specialist promised him an improvement at each visit. But instead he continued to gain weight and to feel worse than before. Curiously, the small group of comrades in misfortune that he had met in the waiting room of the medicine man with the diplomas was shrinking as the months went by. By 1974 they were all new faces. But what had become of the five or six old acquaintances? When Florian M finally realized that they were all in the cemetery, he took definitive leave of Dame Medicine.

A first treatment with acupuncture sedated the pains and brought about a remarkable stabilization of the lupus. The superficial energetic balance was in fact excellent on the day of his first visit to my office. But acupuncture is a medicine of the etheric body. Only an extremely elevated vibratory technique can attain the desired goal of correcting the spatiotemporal deformations of the astral body.

First, my treatment comprised removal of the enormous iatrogenic liability accumulated over 35 years of overvaccination and chemical medication. This went on from April 1980 to July 1981 when the first successes became apparent. My patient could once again take normal baths since his skin was no longer covered by horrible oozing sores. The nephrotic syndrome affecting his kidneys with an important loss of albumin was diminished and his general health was excellent.

I spent the following year in a first genetic regulation following my usual technique which I call the EI cycle. (I will reveal the secret to you later.) The patient was worn out by the massive blows of these constitutional remedies, but felt that life was worth a certain amount of sacrifice. At the September equinox in 1982 I started the treatment of the EII cycle, which is much more powerful, and I finished my work at the summer solstice of 1983. Four years after the beginning of my sequential therapy, and despite certain major additional disappointments, Florian M was cheerfully going about his many activities as a successful businessman.

Case 6.

My sixth presentation touches upon a subject that is not usually treated by internists, since serious psychosomatic illness is usually relegated to the psychiatric trashcan when the mental symptoms become too obvious. On 23 June 1981 a troubled M and Mme P arrived at my office to show me their 15-year-old daughter Mireille who had been anorexic since February. The young lady, an excellent student, had had certain problems at school during the winter. In January a menstrual period had been missed, and there had not been once since. In February a bad flu had dragged on over several weeks causing exhausting night-time perspiration. Although minimized by the family doctor, the fact was that ever since this incident the young girl had stopped eating. She quickly lost a lot of weight and it became obvious that her illness now had to be given the dreaded name of 'anorexia nervosa'.

This illness has killed many young women and will continue to do so as long as the half-doctors continue to believe themselves alone able to treat it. Luckily, a few real doctors have taken the time since Antiquity to observe the surprising relationships that link our feelings to our digestion. I remind you of my first shock in 1968 upon accidentally discovering the work of Dr Victor Pauchet during my military life. I was therefore not very surprised when Dr Senn spoke to us several years later of his interesting research into intestinal flora following the lead of the great German and English precursors. The Swiss researcher devoted 14 pages of his course to the role of 'toxi-infection' in the appearance of all mental illness. Experimentation has proven him correct, since the homoeopath's classical autovaccine cure prepared from the intestinal germs of the patient generally brings about a spectacular improvement in mental character and balance.

The treatment is controversial however, since it is not without risk and must be carried out with caution. The most difficult area is the choice of the appropriate moment for the vaccinal intervention. My teacher, a laboratory man rather than a theoretician, started the autovaccinal process as soon as his ohmmeter indicated the presence of serious 'barriers' that can be identified using Voll's technique. But, as we have seen, Voll's process is not completely trustworthy and can lead to major mistakes owing to a serious misunderstanding of the important elements of the destabilizing sequence. Personally I prefer to prescribe an autovaccinal cure when my sequential treatment has come to the end of all the marking events of my patient's life. It would take too long to explain the reasons for this here, but experience has always proven this approach to be correct.

So I started Mireille's treatment with the usual string of natural or anti-iatrogenic nosodes: Tuberculinum humanum, then BCG (the young girl had managed to have a perfect primary tubercular infection despite the stupid vaccination), Morbillinum, Varicellinum, then Ignatia and Nux vomica, followed by Rubeolinum in February 1982, Vaccinotoxinum in March and DTPP in May. This chronological cleaning itself produced a spectacular improvement in her overall condition. She still wasn't eating normally, but her weight had increased from 35 to 42kg. Her energetic balance was perfect on all 12 control meridians.

I therefore decided to have the autovaccination prepared using a culture of pathogenic germs identified from analysis of a stool sample. The microbic intestinal flora was dominated by a very harmful association of atypical colibaccilli and pyocyanic bacilli that is fairly characteristic of this 'mental' illness. The treatment began, and the young girl had to resign herself to drinking a few drops of the solution each morning in progressively increasing doses. Starting at the September equinox, I began parallel treatment with the EI cycle of genetic correction, which ended at the summer equinox of June 1983. At her last visit on 3 August 1983, Mireille was once again a happy and healthy young lady. The anorexia nervosa was an unpleasant memory of the past.

The therapeutic schema is the same for epilepsy, paranoia, schizophrenia and the severe endogenic depressions, which are among the worst scourges of suffering humankind. I am considered crazy myself when I claim to be able to cure these things without too much difficulty using my sequential therapy coupled with intestinal autovaccination. Yet this is absolutely true, as each of the aforementioned illnesses has given me the occasion to verify the undoubted superiority of Real Medicine.

My teacher states that he has cured many patients whom psychiatrists have declared 'incurable' by using autovaccination coupled with the precarious Voll technique. Unfortunately for those suffering from these illnesses, he has never published the details of his clinical experiments. Even the smallest empirical contribution is welcome if it can help medicine free itself from the pseudoscientific yoke imposed on it by the melancholy 'father of psychiatry'. It is in fact obvious that mental illness doesn't exist! 'Psychiatric' problems come solely from the conflict of biophysical energies that were recognized thousands of years ago and which are very elegantly tamed by astral, etheric, neuroendocrine, toxi-intestinal or mere dietary techniques.

A new tendency has appeared in the United States that finally supports (30 years late) the opinion expressed here. I am referring to the research of Dr Carl C Pfeiffer, founder of the Brain Bio Center of the neuropsychiatric institute of New Jersey, which is moving the therapy of 'mental' illnesses in the direction indicated in 1968(!) by the brilliant, twice winner of the Nobel Prize, Linus Pauling, the inventor of orthomolecular medical philosophy. This new orientation is encouraging since it at last puts the accent on the primacy of the energetic side of the vital process, shown here by the biological catalysis that has been studied with the utmost scientific discipline. While Pfeiffer's experiments are certainly not on the same energetic plane as Real Medicine, they are in the same direction and I consider this to be a good sign.

Case 7.

With my seventh presentation, I will leave the muddy shores of psychosomatics and bring you back to the firm footing of physical realities. A fall on one's back can be very painful and have consequences that make themselves felt years later. At least that is how Fritz S, a young Viennese cook, felt as he complained about the low back pain that he was still experiencing long after he had fallen on the slippery tiles of his kitchen floor. Unfortunately for him the doctors' opinions were slightly different, since the X-rays and lab tests indicated the existence of Bechterew's illness. This awful, creeping form of rheumatism strikes young men and transforms them over the years into stiff, twisted marionettes. I received this sad information one morning in February 1981 by telephone from a friend, who as manager of one of the great Palace hotels of Vienna was worried about his cook and hoping that I could perform a miracle. Unfortunately the diagnosis could not be put in doubt since it came from the equally prestigious university clinic where I had worked 20 years earlier.

I will spare you the details of my treatment. You now know that the only thing required is the correction of the immaterial sequels of major iatrogenic or childhood shocks through chronologically rigorous isotherapy. Vital energy then returns to its previous majestic path. After spending a year in this first clean-up, the vertebral articulations of the young man rapidly stopped suffering. I had at the outset scrapped the eternal anti-inflammatories of illustrious ex-teachers, replacing them advantageously with certain medicinal teas, 'devil's claws' (Harpagophytum) and pineapple enzymes. The cook continued to suffer somewhat from his back during the second phase of my sequential treatment, the difficult EI cycle, but the next correction, the irresistible EII, banished the frightening image of Bechterew to the category of bad memories. As a thank you for curing him, the cook offered me the joy of an identical success in applying the same treatment to his brother, who also suffered from this illness.

Case 8.

Here is another incurable and interesting (in other words horrible) illness that doctors have treated for too long with their usual arrogance, given that its psychosomatic origins were unanimously agreed upon by the faculty. I am speaking of the extremely painful Crohn's disease, also known as terminal ileitis, which ravages the end of the small intestine, and sometimes the colon, with burning and bleeding. It exhausts its victims through frequent and often bloody diarrhoea with a profound effect on their morale that will come as no surprise to you now that you are aware of the close intestinal–psychological link.

Since immunologists have found an interesting aetiological trail, doctors are unable to continue mistaking effects for causes, and the terrible Crohn's disease, become less 'psy', has acquired its scientific letters of nobility. But the causal diagnosis of the faculty isn't worth very much, because it doesn't lead to any kind of curative treatment.

I recognized the enormity of my task in accepting the case in January 1982 of Mme Juliana S, from Budapest, who immigrated to Switzerland after the events in Hungary. The anamnesis was difficult and confused, with many missing dates and destabilizing shocks: pneumonia, operations, mumps, scarlet fever, measles, all kinds of vaccinations, dysfunctional kidneys, amoebae, enormous psychological shocks, cortisone treatments, chemical battering ... The diagnosis had been made in Switzerland in 1981, after some hesitation, by the university medical clinic where Juliana S was employed. It was later confirmed by the specialist responsible for her treatment and by the classical clinical evolution of the case.

I was somewhat discouraged by the confusion of the initial facts so important to the success of my treatment. The energetic imbroglio was extreme and the severity of the ailment was terrible to observe. But her vital energy didn't appear to be too diminished, and the spatiotemporal breaking point had not yet been reached.

Because of the specialist and his high doses of cortisone, I lost precious time in correcting the iatrogenic imbalance. I then put together an acceptable therapeutic sequence which was extremely tiring for the patient. The success achieved was beyond my hopes. The diarrhoea and intestinal pain rapidly lost their habitual violence even though from the outset my patient courageously gave up all the chemical protection proposed by the gastroenterologist. After a year of chronological correction carried out with the irreplaceable help of radiesthesia, I was finally able in January 1983 to introduce my genetically directed sequences, which stabilize the morbid constitution. The three or four minor alerts that still occur annually are overcome with common homoeopathic remedies, and the future now seems less sinister.

Naturally the allopaths curious enough to read my book won't miss the opportunity to point out that Crohn's disease (like the seven other scourges that I mentioned above) often evolves in phases that can periodically involve welcome periods of remission and even an occasional complete recovery. I agree, but then how does one explain that it is always my patients who recover 'spontaneously'? Why do my allopathic colleagues so rarely experience the wonderful joys of these unhoped-for recoveries? An explanation for this curiosity would certainly interest the general public. Luckily, more and more patients seek information, compare things and finally discover by themselves that the only real doctors are the ones that heal. And they don't hesitate to choose those doctors over all other therapists be they a hundred times more knowledgeable, charming or enterprising. My ninth and last story will demonstrate this.

Case 9.

On 9 February 1982 I received a visit from a very nice woman from Athens who had come seeking advice concerning her 7-year-old son. The handsome little blond boy that I saw in the photograph didn't look ill at all, and yet his life had been poisoned since infancy by dramatic episodes of extremely serious diarrhoea alternated with repeated rhinopharynx and bronchial infections. Since the child had come close to death several times, the Athenian doctors had recommended that the parents seek advice from a highly reputed foreign doctor. Their choice fell upon Professor R, who was unquestionably the most famous paediatrician in my country. This brilliant technician's combination of keen intelligence with encyclopedic knowledge has my admiration.

Little Nils was then hospitalized for the first time in the spring of 1978 and a diagnosis was made: immune deficiency due to dysgamma-globulinaemia. In other words, the child defended himself poorly in cases of infection because he lacked the requisite quantity of certain indispensable blood proteins. I went through the interesting and very complete file brought by the mother and saw that neither the first hospitalization nor the subsequent ones had managed to find the key to the mystery. Why was this occurring? The professor gave no answer. His entire science amounted to providing the laboratory result. But the child was in danger and had to be cared for. Nothing simpler! Since he lacks gamma-globulin, let's inject him with it from time to time and everything will be fine. Easy!

After 3 long years of treatment, Nils' parents finally understood the truth. (The child was receiving from one to three muscular injections a month of the precious gamma-globulin he needed. If the injections were less frequent, the virulence of the infectious germs returned.) Putting an end to this war that was at a standstill, the mother decided on a more dynamic tactic and made the trip to Lausanne.

The little Athenian's treatment was child's play! The correct diagnosis was made immediately: a commonplace sequence of destabilizing events where dehydration and the sequels of an old concussion had further worsened the usual iatrogenic vaccinal shocks. I started treatment without even seeing the patient, asking the mother to give him the first three small packets of the remedy which was chronologically indicated. I saw the child for the first time on 26 February 1982. The Lung–Large Intestine energetic imbalance was completely obvious. It was a case for a beginner! I gave the mother the next three remedies of my corrective sequence and we made an appointment for 5 July.

Nils had made tremendous progress. The rhinitis, cough and sinusitis had disappeared. Since our first appointment he had only received one injection of the costly gamma-globulin for a severe diarrhoea accompanied by vomiting. The osteopathic treatment I had prescribed for the old head wound had also done a lot of good. I continued the chronological treatment with two commonplace doses and saw Nils again in September for the final corrective shock for the severe traumatism, which had taken place at 3 months of age (cerebral concussion with epidural haematoma). I started the intestinal autovaccinal cure and my EI cycle of genetic correction simultaneously, and an appointment was fixed for February 1983 to complete the treatment. By then the child was superb and no longer required any gamma-globulin. He had recovered a perfect energetic balance and was cured.

I saw him 1 year later for a check-up, and he had not been seriously ill since our last visit. His vital energy had recovered the serene dignity of his innocent age. This spectacular recovery glaringly reveals the two directions we can give to our destiny when illness strikes head on. On the one hand there is the imposing official direction with its parade of white gowns, the knowledge of its scholars, its costly research, repeated blood tests, numerous injections, accumulation of travel, hotel/hospital/doctor and pharmaceutical bills. In addition there is the tiresome, restrictive, costly and unsatisfying treatment that comes with it, not to mention the uncertainty for the future and the growing dependence on the all-powerful medical profession.

On the other hand, there is the elegance and conciseness of Real Medicine. The simplicity of its approach makes it available to anyone in good faith. It gives them more power than erudition, technique and chemistry combined.

The story of little Nils is exemplary in the clarity of the verdict it hands down.

SEVENTEEN

The failures

In fairness to the reader and to scientific honesty, I am duty bound to provide a complete account of all aspects of Real Medicine. A cold shower is sometimes necessary to prevent the imagination running away with itself after the euphoria of unhoped-for medical victories. Sequential therapy is not a cure-all and cannot always be used. The reasons for mistakes are numerous and the failures can tarnish its radiance and create doubt concerning its unique efficiency. To avoid any misunderstanding, this chapter will review the multiple causes of failure, and the deceptive traps into which beginners will inevitably fall, be they half-doctors or experienced homoeopaths.

DIET

First, it must be categorically stated that no medicine can achieve lasting results if the patient's diet is not healthy. This initial requirement, brilliantly formulated by Hippocrates, was put aside in some dark corner of history for centuries. The dietetics taught in our faculties today is a pale caricature of the royal science which like health, should occupy the key professorial chairs in our universities. It is not, however, through counting calories or joules, nor by inventorying proteins and carbohydrates, that students will learn to give their future patients the solid foundation from which life will spring. One must not forget that life is born of life, and that the food of our physical bodies, as miserable as this destination may be, must also respect the superior spatiotemporal continuum, which rules over our destinies. The vibrations of the nutritive molecular constituents must be perfectly synchronized with those of our cellular constituents in order to fit harmoniously into the great space–time continuum, which defines our life.

This is the price of health. If a doctor peremptorily announces to you that your diet plays no role in the evolution of your illness, he deserves to lose your confidence immediately, even if he is a renowned professor. Unfortunately they are legion, these plenipotentiary specialists who counsel our governments about health and make lawful the sifting of flour and the refining of sugars, salt or rice. These same all-powerful experts are responsible for the criminal delays in anticancer research through their preference, to the great benefit of the merchants, for chemo- and radiotherapy.

To my knowledge no Western university medical school provides a dietetics course deserving of the name. Worse, the precursors and honest scholars are ridiculed, if not attacked outright. A local example of this is our university's pedantic and negative opinion on the remarkable work carried out by Dr Catherine Kousmine in the nearby town of Lutry. She acquired an international reputation for her extremely satisfying results in treating multiple sclerosis and other degenerative illnesses. These surprising successes were primarily obtained through an extremely severe reform of the patient's diet. The recipe for her famous 'Budwig cream' is distributed by all healthfood stores and used every morning by thousands of enthusiastic followers. During my hospital internships in Lausanne, this great lady was mentioned only with contempt (it has been a long time since doctors were gentlemen!), but the indefensible behaviour of my colleagues could not prevent a growing public from following the evening courses that she gave or applying her dietetic precepts. Sick and well alike have been reinvigorated in this way, and I take advantage of the opportunity here offered me to recommend her books highly.

Yet while it is true that Real Medicine cannot be conceived without a rigorous change in our alimentation it must be said that this is not in itself enough to reinstate the lost balance of vital energy totally confused by a long series of destabilizing shocks. In fact many of the patients I have seen had followed Dr Kousmine's instructions to the letter and had still not recovered their health.

It was only after I had been able to identify the energetic imbroglio and correct it with my sequential therapy that I could re-establish the energetic balance of these patients and proclaim them cured.

There is no stable recovery except through the spatiotemporal realignment of the thread of our lives. This is why chronic illnesses that are tamed by macrobiotic or other dietetic means inevitably reappear at the slightest lapse in alimentary discipline. Dr Kousmine elegantly points this out in her books, as do other pioneers of healthy nutrition. Another famous example is that of Dr A Sattilaro of Philadelphia who cured himself of an advanced cancer with a macrobiotic diet, and described in his book *Recalled by Life* the harm caused immediately by any deviation from it.

Sequential therapy and dietetics therefore appear to be indissociably linked, since both are indispensable to the precious state of balance that defines health. If the second is unquestionably inferior to the first (because tied to the inferior spatiotemporal continuum), it is none the less the second fundamental pillar of a medicine that heals. I am conscious of its enormous importance, which would justify a parenthesis as large as this book. But other people have also recognized this fact, and you will have no trouble finding numerous works devoted to healthy diet, that essential discipline censured by the faculty.

If real therapists generally manage to avoid this first trap of guilty ignorance regarding dietetics it is often thanks to their patients, given that the general public is much better informed than the medical profession about the dangers of overrefined and devitalized industrial food. Most patients who have removed themselves from the palliative care of a doctor have generally taken the trouble to eliminate white bread, white sugar, hot-pressed oils, industrial preserves and other such wonders of our decadent civilization from their diets. The universal obsession with weight control has put fashion for once on the right side of things. Luckily the prestige of the faculty, this eternal latecomer, can no longer counteract the immense powers of persuasion of the media, open to a vast public.

OSTEOPATHIC LESIONS

There is, however, a second trap into which a beginner does risk falling even if he is a complete doctor. Remember the first pages of this book in which I often admitted that despite the excellence of my biological weapons, I had been unable to stop the progress of certain chronic ailments. Unaware of Voll's less-than-perfect theory of blockages, I had sometimes thought that these failures could be attributed to an energetic blockage of vertebral origin. I had without knowing it put my finger on the most important cause of failure in Real Medicine: osteopathic lesions.

Since the enormous range of osteopathy is still little known in Europe, and especially in my country, I think it appropriate to give a brief introduction to this major art that is a hundred years old and is the indispensable third pillar of Real Medicine. Like homoeopathy, this brilliant discipline, which was invented in 1874 by the American Andrew Taylor Still, is not taught at our universities. I first heard of it in the famous 'Readings' of the well-known American visionary Edgar Cayce, and then from my aunt Mlle Ginette Elmiger who was a pioneer in manual techniques. Dr Senn had wanted to introduce it in his courses at the Cornelius Celsus Foundation, but unfortunate obstacles didn't allow his students to benefit from such an opportunity, unique in Switzerland, to learn this essential discipline systematically disparaged by our medical authorities.

Luckily the publication in September 1983 of a remarkable work by Lionelle and Marielle Issartel *L'Ostéopathie Exactement*, is now available to fill this inadmissible gap in the education of young doctors. They will be more than a little surprised that once again the medicine of tomorrow is being learned at the local bookshop and not on the benches of a classroom.

I will try to summarize briefly the fundamental aspects of this doctrine. The inventor, Dr Still, developed his new concept from two Greek words for 'bones' and 'sickness'. He had noticed that certain clinical signs could be tied to certain incorrect positions of the articular surfaces. Even a slight disturbance of the free interplay of the articulations could cause the appearance in another part of the body of an illness that was apparently unrelated to the articular problem. Naturally, the induced problem was more significant if the mistreated articular surfaces belonged to the major structural category of bones.

The main structural base of our skeleton is the spinal column, and it is the osteopathic lesions of the backbone that are the cause of the most common complaints. By studying the complete picture of the disorder that was created, the skeletal malpositioning and the reactional modalities of the corrective manipulations, Still deduced three fundamental principles, which are the substance of his therapeutic technique.

This trilogy is summarized by the Issartel sisters in the following key concepts: the structural unity of the body, the subjugation of physiological functions to the integrity of structures, and self-healing due to the functional impetus after correction of the structural alteration. What links these three terms and makes their interaction possible is necessarily a force. But what is this power that underlies the complex tangle of structures and functions? You have probably guessed: it is our old friend vital energy, whose first physical expression will shortly be described.

By directing his attention to the complex pathology of vertebral problems, Dr Still rediscovered an ancient truth of the art of healing that had been long forgotten. He had discovered the principal channel of this force of life, the privileged vector that the Ancients quite simply called the 'tree of life', that supple and hollow pillar that is the receptacle of the commanding keyboard that electronics will never be able to imitate. Bone marrow is to vital energy what conducting wire is to electricity. Its material integrity and that of its relation to our overall structures is indispensable to the harmonious flow of our lives. By correcting the tiny displacements of the mechanical structure, Still broadened the field open to the impetuous flow of vital energy, powerful but too subtle to withstand the slightest physical obstacle to its movement.

You have probably noticed the analogy between the osteopathic approach and the sequential therapy: the unique goal of both is the liberation of vital energy from destabilizing constraints. Only the level of intervention is different. With the first, the liberating action is physical and spatial, close to the lower continuum. With the second it is solely immaterial and more temporal.

CRANIAL LESIONS

Dr Still was a pioneer. But it was only after his brilliant successor Dr William Garner Sutherland made his major discovery that osteopathy became the wonderful therapeutic instrument that we know today. Sutherland, who studied Still's osteopathy at the beginning of the century, had been fascinated by an anatomical detail of the cranial bones that was not mentioned by his teachers. The cranial surfaces have a surprising characteristic: they are bevelled. Fifty years after American osteopathy, and like tens of thousands of other medical students standing at their dissecting tables and holding the bones that make up the skull, I also noticed this peculiarity. At the time, like everyone else, I also asked the obvious question: why? And the professor gave the classical reply: the bevel increases the area of the attached bone surfaces thus improving the solidity of the cranial sutures. If my teacher had read Sutherland's *The Cranial Bowl*, he would have given me the correct answer instead, and I would perhaps have become an osteopath and not a doctor.

The answer comes solely from Sutherland's genius and like all brilliant solutions it is obvious in its simplicity. The cranial sutures are bevelled because they are articulations and not sutures. Let me explain. The bones of the skull are very thin strips assembled side by side. If the sutures of this assemblage were cut at right angles, the slightest increase in cranial volume would automatically cause the dislocation of the skull. Instead, since the contact surfaces are enlarged by the bevel, the same increase in internal volume only causes a gentle sliding of the two overlapping surfaces which form the articulation. Since the sutures aren't rigid, the dilation of the contents is easily absorbed by the elasticity of the container.

Yes, this is really Sutherland's most fantastic discovery: the skull is not a rigid and solid sphere; it pulsates! And why does it pulsate? Because the brain itself pulsates! It possesses a rhythmic movement of expansion and contraction at a rate of 10 to 14 beats a minute. Sutherland discovered this phenomenon and named it the 'primary respiratory mechanism' (PRM) by analogy with the pulmonary respiratory rhythm, which is of the same frequency but cannot be superimposed. Naturally, 'scientific' minds deny the existence of this phenomenon, because only an exceptional sensitivity acquired during a long apprenticeship allows this extraordinary perception. For decades doctors have ridiculed osteopaths, treating them as charlatans. But recently this arrogance has had to give way. As a result of progress in electronics, this tiny beating can now be measured. It even seems that the brain of a foetus has a pulse well in advance of that of the heart, as the minute study of intrauterine films apparently proves. And so this brilliant precursor was as close as one can get to the truth, and he thus concretized Still's intuitions by localizing the first physical motor of the complex energetic network that links functions to structures.

And now we must dare the big questions. What is this force that animates our brain? Where does it come from? You know the answer as well as I do: it can only be vital energy in its most material formal manifestation. Coming from above, it needs this first condenser, our brain, to adapt its subtle vibrations to our lowly physical condition. Of all the space–time clusters that impose themselves on the lower continuum, Sutherland's primary respiratory mechanism is clearly the one most directly accessible to our senses. Trained hands can easily feel this wave of life pulsate in all parts of the body. Its strongest propagation is most easily perceived along the 'tree of life' where it flows from the head to the sacrum, that last solid mass of the spine, which acts as a buffer sending the emitted wave back to the brain.

One can easily imagine that the propagation of such a subtle pulsing wave inevitably encounters certain mishaps in the course of a lifetime. The main risk, which is inherent to the binary nature of all energetic manifestations, is the loss of the Yin–Yang balance through impact with another energy. Such traumatizing events, to which the osteopaths were the first to attribute a destabilizing significance, are all too frequent. Here is a short list, which is already enough to provide food for thought.

The first risk is that of birth. And here a brief parenthesis is necessary to denounce one of the most terrible aberrations in the history of medicine. For centuries, and in all civilizations, women gave birth in a squatting or kneeling position. This is the natural position and requires flexibility and genuine vigour. With a lesser physical condition, as was the case over time with inactive and wealthy women, help was required in the form of either manual support or obstetric chairs. But the position remained vertical. The height of refinement was reached in the 17th century at the

French court, where the royal obstetrician decided that the elegant beauties of the court would be put to bed to avoid tiring them. This prestigious idiot's decree was to have incalculable consequences on all of Western civilization. The stupid fashion spread from Versailles to the other European courts and then to the entire world, finally imposing itself as the only way to have children.

Unfortunately it's true, ladies. No medical student learns any other way to deliver a child. I'm honestly surprised that doctors haven't convinced you to try to defecate while lying down since it's so much more restful! Anyone can grasp the incongruity of such a proposal, yet it's an identical ineptitude that the faculty has been proposing for 3 centuries.

By placing the parturiants in a prone position, the obstetricians provoke a series of negative events that transform the natural act into a medical one, grotesque and artificial. Childbirth no longer occurs without physical or chemical help: labour is prolonged or artificially shortened, induced labour is often inadequate, the contractions are too violent and the expulsion is no longer spontaneous and requires pulling by the head, often with forceps or other equipment. And what becomes of the newborn's skull in this adventure?

Still and Sutherland's followers have demonstrated beyond any doubt that most cranial osteopathic lesions are obstetric in nature. To these must be added later deformations following a shock: a fall on the head or on the tailbone (a kick in the behind is not less harmful than an outright slap in the face), a slip on stairs, etc. The shock can also be spread over several years, disguised as a permanent constraint. I'm referring here to the ugly braces that orthodontists attach to misaligned teeth, once again treating the effects instead of the causes. This practice is all the rage here, while in the United States (from where the fashion came, with the customary delay), osteopaths seem to have convinced a growing public that the force moving the teeth out of line is merely a pathological deviation of the primary respiratory mechanism. To put the teeth back in the right place before the age of 7, it is often necessary only to have an osteopath 'remodel' the child's skull. A few sessions of tiny manipulations with the hands are enough, and the result is unbelievable. If the primary respiratory mechanism chose the teeth as a way out, this was precisely in response to the law of least resistance. Teeth are only attached by their buried pole; their free pole can move without too much harm and evacuate (like a lightning rod) the deviated celestial energies. If the dentist creates too strong a resistance to this escape route, the diverted cranial energy will do its damage elsewhere. One cannot go against the laws of nature with impunity.

* * *

This very hasty overview of the most innovative medical discipline next to homoeopathy was necessary. It will have helped the reader to understand that the energetic balance of perfect health cannot be achieved as long as the most tangible manifestation of vital energy is not harmoniously balanced. It is impossible to count the number of homoeopathic treatments, properly carried out, even isosequential, that have failed owing to a misunderstanding of osteopathic lesions or to the impossibility of their correction. I particularly want to warn Voll's followers who, finding 'blockage' during the ohmmetric examination, will attribute the energetic imbalance to an old illness or even a constitutional defect, while the cause is simply a common osteopathic lesion. This frequent and dangerous mistake of interpretation can destroy an entire life. Be careful!

But even if it is true that the best homoeopathic treatment in the world is inadequate to reinstate an equilibrium that has been disturbed by a deviation of the primary respiratory mechanism, it is also true that the best osteopath in the world will not be able to restore health if the patient is caught up in an energetic imbroglio located at the superior immaterial level. Additionally, the osteopaths in whom I have confidence have always told me that their treatments were much more rapidly efficient with my patients than with patients sent by doctors who were less familiar with chronological isotherapy.

Thus osteopathy, like dietetics, remains dependent on sequential therapy, the unique leader of Real Medicine.

LOSS OF TIME

A third cause of failure that is common to all techniques of energetic readaptation is their late start. The fact is that patients often seek the care of real doctors only once they have gone through innumerable toxic and useless palliative treatments that the medicine of officialdom and banks has authoritatively imposed. This systematic chemical hammering not only adds a serious intoxication to the initial destabilization, suppressing the few reactional abilities of an overloaded organism, but it also causes a loss of precious time: the time spent in useless poisoning and the time needed by the therapist to eliminate the sequels of this poisoning. And by stupidly wasting time in this manner, the patient can finally miss his ultimate meeting with Time: the infamous spatiotemporal breaking point beyond which it is useless to expect a reactional adaptation.

It would be easy for me to present here a gloomy sequence of those desperate cases where despite my best efforts I have been unable to re-establish a balance lost for ever by having gone beyond the breaking point. I prefer instead to give my readers this somewhat solemn advice: go to see a real doctor while there is still time! Personally I find nothing more difficult than to have to refuse the pressing requests of patients with severe chronic illnesses who have been atrociously let down by orthodox medicine. I receive moving cries for help, but I know at the outset that my art will be useless when I read in their letters that they have 'tried everything with no results for ten or twenty years'. For these poor people who are often also burdened with the weight of age, only palliative relief is possible, and my immaterial techniques would have no effect.

This doesn't mean that Real Medicine is inaccessible to the elderly. I have often had the pleasure of successfully going through an excellent sequential therapy with older people who felt all the better for it. But they had all had the wisdom to lead a life without excess and had always viewed doctor's pills with the prudence that the name imposes: *pharmakon*, poison!

OTHER CAUSES OF FAILURE

These classical stumbling blocks explain the vast majority of our failures. When a patient spends his life misusing alimentary hygiene, closing his eyes to flaws in posture or of the skull, seeking the easy palliative solution to a chronic problem, he can no longer expect to recover health without making severe sacrifices plus intelligent thought and sagacity on the part of the real doctor he has chosen as guide. But a doctor is only a man, and he can also make mistakes. If he has never heard of Voll's mesenchymatous blockages, and if he doesn't use nosodes, he will only obtain the incomplete results to which traditional homoeopathy and acupuncture have accustomed their adepts.

If the homoeopath is stuck in a classical attitude, strictly Kentist for example (Kent only gave the one remedy indicated by the immediate clinical picture), he will merely be able to move his patients forward with a little hop at each appointment, instead of giving them the giant's boots that are needed to catch up with Time.

If the doctor has heard too much about Voll's barriers, he risks a different mistake in blindly following his machine. In Chapter 6 you saw a demonstration of the typical error that I have called the 'Mikado effect'. This mistake is made daily by those who imitate Voll but who have been unable to refine their own sensitivity and acquire enough wisdom to respect the rigorous chronology imposed by Hering.

Just like my teacher who kept a pile of his illustrious 'unicist' colleagues' shamefully 'pluralist' prescriptions on his desk, I have saved a group of files showing the failures of my Vollian colleagues, be they the students or the master himself. The list of these mistakes would be too technical to interest the public. The main error is always a violation of the Law through neglect of an essential detail, unrecognized, forgotten or simply underestimated. I have carefully saved this documentary material for the edification of those who will follow me, since one often learns the most from failures. I am not doing this out of spite, and hope to retain enough humility and humour to withstand the criticism of the first innovator who will find the flaw in my sequential method.

To bring to an end the list of mistakes that can be imputed to doctors themselves, I must draw the attention of students as well as their future patients to the essential quality that a therapist must have: moderation. Yes, it is generally because of a blatant lack of restraint that a doctor fails in his endeavour. One must not forget that the homoeopathic potency is a 'force', in other words a concentrate of immaterial energy with a very broad range of action. If the doctor uses high potencies, he must recognize that these seemingly harmless little pills are real 'bombs'. Dear reader, beware of homoeopaths who use very high potencies too frequently!

To illustrate this warning here is a last story, bitter and funny, which almost turned into a tragedy owing to the clumsy impetuosity of an inexperienced colleague.

Since the age of 12 years, Mme F M (from Cheseaux-sur-Lausanne) had been treated by my first teacher, who in 20 years of treatment (waged with many bombs) had been unable to stabilize her constitution, which was seriously burdened with hereditary tuberculosis. Unable to see her in 1974, I sent her to a young colleague who was also a student of the same teacher, but who emigrated to the United States shortly thereafter. The treatment was then taken up by a third doctor, who correctly identified the constitutional problem and decided to correct it right away with one of the major remedies in our pharmacopoeia: Phosphorus. Since small doses of this dangerous metalloid didn't bring about the expected results, he made the terrible mistake of prescribing stronger and stronger potencies. When he had finally given the 50,000th Korsakovian potency, the drama exploded.

The anxiety that had been haunting the patient for more than 20 years came to life with such violence under this terrible shock that the poor woman tried to kill herself. This fatal act was precluded by a friend's presence of mind and the immediate termination of this imprudent colleague's treatment for whom this was not the first major blunder. The young woman whom I saw on an emergency basis that October morning in 1980 was a miserable wreck, and sad evidence of the mockery that had been made of a wonderful medicine. I had enormous difficulty in convincing the family not to take legal action and in dissuading the furious (and violent) husband from trying to kill my predecessor. It took me more than 3 years, and a lot of persuasive energy, finally to re-establish the confused equilibrium. But the intense resentment of the victim was calmed only by the intervention of a well-known clairvoyant from Paris. At first glance, and without knowing anything about what had taken place, the prophetess pronounced sentence: 'You are in quite a state, little lady! Do you know the law of Karma? Yes? Well everything that is happening to you is your own fault! You were a doctor in another life, and a bad doctor, more attached to money and prestige than to the well-being of your patients. Your punishment is to now suffer in your own flesh the suffering inflicted by another bad doctor.' The young woman laughed wholeheartedly in telling me this uncommon diagnosis, which she willingly accepted since she was quite used to the audacious reasoning of oriental philosophies.

This overview of technical errors must not allow us to forget the other important source of failure, attributable to the attitude of the patients themselves. Every year I record defections caused by the faintheartedness of those seeking help but who demand an immediate recovery without having the patience to suffer a little bit to achieve their objective. They do not want to understand that a long series of shocks to the energetic balance can't be erased without the victim reliving 'backwards', in a lesser way, the problems that this litany of shocks created. The most timid are frightened by the violence which the liberating isopathic impact can have. They lose confidence and return straight away to the preceding doctor who, knowing only half of the medical art, hastens to deride the other half. One can't blame the patient, who is free to choose, but this misunderstanding of the intimate mechanisms of isosequential healing is none the less very disappointing. I hope that this book will help to dissipate some of this confusion!

Often this Real Medicine is destined to fail because of the controversy that it creates within families. The husband, generally more materialist–rationalist than the wife, decides that he is against the principle of immateriality. If his wife doesn't stand up to him, the treatment won't be enthusiastically followed, and will even be abandoned at the slightest beneficial homoeopathic 'aggravation'. If in addition the medical expenses aren't reimbursed by medical health care insurance policies it is a sure-fire condemnation, since money often counts more than health.

It is unfortunately becoming increasingly difficult to practise real medicine in our industrialized countries, and in mine in particular. A certain heroic spirit is required of both the doctor and his patients, since the opposition is strong. The all powerful pharmaceutical lobby, which controls important pawns in the game of politics, is determined to put us down. In Lausanne we have also recently been the object of a painful boycott organized by the 'Federation of Medical Insurances', which is unable to tolerate the idea of freedom in medical practice. Together with the few rare doctors who have remained independent, we lost a first legal proceeding against the Federation and are anxiously awaiting the appeal verdict. Is medicine still a liberal profession? I have to say that the prognosis is gloomy.

We are terribly alone and very weak compared with this coalition of opposing forces. We can't even count on the spiritual aid of the major established religions. On the contrary, certain evangelical tendencies are increasing the ranks of our enemies. It is not uncommon that I receive letters cancelling appointments and arguing an incompatibility between Real Medicine (which apparently is manipulating satanic forces!) and 'commitment to the Christian faith'. One of my friends and neighbours gave me a recently published brochure that attacked homoeopathy and radiesthesia in a tone which bore no small resemblance to that of the Inquisition. He had received it for his edification from the vicar of the local parish who was horrified to learn that he was an adept of our art.

Even though I could easily take this attitude from another age as an attack against my convictions, I can still provide a lesson in tolerance to these sectarian opponents by forgiving them their intransigence.

PART THREE

CONSTITUTIONAL ILLNESSES
Complete sequential therapy

EIGHTEEN

The four predispositions

The fact that Hahnemannian medicine derives great benefit from the study of constitutions will not be contested by anyone. From the outset knowledgeable critics of this new method recognized the enormous advantage represented by these diagnostic criteria, which encompass a first appreciation of the hereditary predispositions. In addition, and even more interesting, is the immediate improvement of the flawed constitution that occurs with the administration of a correctly selected remedy. Objective observers have always acknowledged this evident superiority of homoeopathy over its allopathic sister who lacks the ability to regulate heredity. It is to this power that so many brilliant successes must be attributed.

We will now explore in detail this notion of constitutions, so dear to homoeopaths. Readers should be warned that they won't find here a bookish nomenclature of the constitutional types that different schools feel they have identified and which have been described elsewhere in endless detail. The study of constitutions is indeed interesting, but it is of only minor importance in the global appreciation of our genetic patrimony. What I mean by 'constitution' should not be understood in this book as the definition of a substratum with the description of its constituent elements (carbonates, sodium, fluorine, silica, etc). The term that I am using is merely a designation for the unfortunate predisposition of our genetic code, given a hidden flaw, to lead towards one or another morbid symptomatology.

First of all I must point out that this idea of the subordination of health to a condition anterior to birth is as old as medicine itself. It is very much alive today in all of us, and the young mothers entrusting me with their children harmed by overvaccination understand very quickly why this misfortune has struck their offspring instead of other children who underwent the same iatrogenic pollution. It is evident that each of us comes into this world with a different potential for health, even if scientific knowledge is not yet able to measure all the characteristics of this inheritance.

It is once again to the wonderful genius of Samuel Hahnemann that medicine owes its first successful attempt at description and correction of the constitutions. This exceptional observer had noticed that his treatments didn't have the same impact in chronic and in acute illness. In addition, with acute illness the same remedies didn't necessarily produce the same effects. From this he derived the concept of individual sensitivity in the patient, which he rapidly integrated into the more global vision of inherited predispositions. Popular common sense has always recognized that certain terrible illnesses pursue some families and not others, thereby implicitly accepting a type of hereditary transmission. Hahnemann was the first to establish a brief classification of the principal chronic ailments that are attached to different anomalies of the constitution.

Here is another thing that is absolutely evident. Constitutions are not uniformly stable and healthy in everyone. Just like different soils in which plants can grow more or less well, our physical bodies are built following certain more or less favourable criteria from our genetic patrimony. Hahnemann was able to identify the three principal defects of the soil in which we grow. He called them 'psora', 'sycosis' and 'luetism'. As this book is not a treatise on homoeopathy I do not plan to further the study of this famous trilogy. Instead I hope to give you the brief description that is necessary to an intimate understanding of Real Medicine.

PSORA

In his *Discussion of Chronic Illnesses,* Hahnemann provided an analysis of this first predisposition in which he saw the primary origin of most chronic illnesses identified at his time. (Predisposition, sometimes termed 'diathesis', refers to the general tendency of a person to contract a certain type of illness.) Hahnemann called this first constitutional weakness psora after a very widespread illness of his period, the mange (called *psora* in both Latin and Greek). He attributed to the mange, the causal agent of which had not been identified at that time, the characteristic of eliminating the residues of misfunctioning internal organs through the skin. If the doctor impedes the skin's role of elimination through hasty external treatments, the 'cured' skin infection is replaced with far more serious general troubles requiring treatment with internal medicine. The innumerable 'mangy' people of Hahnemann's period (almost all illnesses now encompassed by dermatology were given this name at the time) were powerfully and efficiently 'treated'. Scabby and pockmarked skin was rapidly removed by the corrosive effects of highly toxic ointments. But the unfortunate patient had to pay for this rejuvenation of the skin with crises of gout or asthma, digestive illness, or other afflictions that were taking the place of the 'external' pathology that had been thwarted.

Hahnemann had noticed this sort of balance between internal problems and their external correspondences and the link between the aggravation of one type of problem and the improvement of the other. He had discovered the great Law, which his brilliant disciple Constantine Hering was to have the honour of clearly defining for the first time. In addition, he had the wonderful intuition that many chronic illnesses were merely the expression of the interiorization of this 'mange' that was so widespread in those times of inadequate hygiene. In his treatise on chronic illnesses, Hahnemann provided an impressive list of all the ailments that he suspected were of 'psoric' origin. The list contained almost all the illnesses that are inventoried today under internal medicine! The modern observer can't help but smile at a generalization like this, which would seem obsessional. Yet this brilliant precursor was once again correct, since the treatment invented by his disciple to cure these internal complications brought irrefutable proof of the veracity of his theory: it worked!

And what did Hering invent that was so extraordinary? Like the master, he curbed logical reasoning, preferring the analogical approach. Since the problem is caused by a suppression from the exterior to the interior, recovery can come only from a reversal of this movement. A means had to be found to 'call up' the noxious elements that were inside back up to the skin, thus starting the beneficial reverse movement. Where else to find this impetus but on the skin itself? Hering set about gathering samples of these 'mangy' skins which he then incorporated with the classic universal support, milk sugar, and potentized according to Hahnemann's rules. He called his new remedy Psorinum. This is how the greatest remedy of the new medicine was invented. By giving it systematically to all his patients suffering from psora starting in 1834, he cured chronic catarrh of all kinds, rheumatism, colic, black bile and other congestions with stupefying ease. Yes, Psorinum is truly the greatest of remedies. A century and a half after its invention, it still cures just as surely the innumerable problems for which it is indicated. Modern homoeopaths all over the world prescribe it every day. This masterpiece of the pharmacopoeia has never been outdated although the explanation that scientific minds have given to its active properties has substantially evolved over the years with the changes in medical knowledge. The psoric constitution is no longer considered as the chronic phase of the mange. It now has a more scholarly name: 'neuroarthritic diathesis', more commonly known as allergy.

Homoeopaths currently attribute to Psorinum the function of a bioenergetic starter, a kind of generic signal that can set in motion in a predisposed individual a series of characteristic adaptive reactions. That this cybernetic reaction is linked to the genetic code now seems evident to biologists enamoured of biophysics. In this respect psora is truly a hereditary predisposition, received from one's ancestry and passed on to one's descendants. Like any passive asset, it can be depreciated or can gain in value depending on the investment manager. Ever since Hering, this evolution can be controlled. Psorinum is the key.

SYCOSIS

Another very curious skin disease was quite widespread at the beginning of the 19th century. This affliction, which is very rare today, covered its victim's skin with multiple growths that were fig-shaped (Latin: *ficus*, fig), and which doctors cauterized or removed. Since these growths had a marked tendency to reappear, Hahnemann labelled them a predisposition, which he called sycosis, from *sukon*, the Greek for fig. He rapidly came to the conclusion that this predisposition represented another fundamental part of our ancestral baggage, and he was able to link to it a number of chronic skin and mucous problems. In psora, the initial ailment was the mange. In sycosis, it was the venereal disease gonorrhoea, which was extremely widespread at the time and almost incurable.

You can now imagine how the early homoeopaths found the remedy capable of improving this second constitution. They could have no precise idea of the agent of gonorrhoea since germs were not yet known. So they proceeded as with the mange, simply taking samples of what they saw on the mucus: pus and mucopurulent secretions. Incorporated with milk sugar and potentized, this mixture became the second great remedy of the new medicine and was baptized Medorrhinum from two Greek words meaning 'discharge' and 'genitals'.

Like the preceding remedy, it is not really a nosode since it has not been prepared from the germ of a specific illness. To indicate that it still comes from living things homoeopaths call this kind of remedy a 'biotherapeutic'. Like Psorinum, Medorrhinum cures the innumerable pathological manifestations falling within its range: warts, condylomas, various tumours, chronic mucous or articular irritation, chronic conjunctivitis and urogenital discharge.

Like psora, sycosis has fascinated homoeopaths who have tried to explain it. Today the venereal element is no longer in the forefront although it is still not negligible. Some have considered this constitution the principal factor in the development of cancer, which is not too far from the truth. Sycosis is even sometimes called 'cancerism', but this label can be misleading. Lastly, since the work of the great English homoeopath Dr Burnett, we can attribute to it another essential role – and one with which I fully agree – our reactive mode to vaccinations. We will see later how to interpret this notion of constitutions in an even more modern way by allowing our analogical intuition to roam freely.

LUETISM

The word comes from the Latin *lues*, which means epidemic and matter in liquefaction. Doctors habitually use this term instead of its synonym which is too well known to the public: syphilis. This other important venereal disease was absolutely devastating at Hahnemann's time since doctors could counter it only with derisory treatments. Our great innovator was the first (again!) to notice that syphilis was not an external illness, but one that evolved from inside to outside. By cauterizing the ulcerated sores the problem was merely worsened because it blocked a valuable way out of the body. (This simplistic 'anti' reasoning, so dear to the allopaths, can be found in every epoch.) These wretched treatments created a diverse pathology of various internal problems: neurological illnesses, skeletal pains, vascular and kidney illness, chronic infections of the rhinopharynx, etc.

How to put this mess into some kind of order? The answer came from another application of analogical thought: the homeopath corrects the luetic constitution by prescribing the biotherapeutic Luesinum, which is made from the vile mass of liquefied flesh taken directly from the syphilis sore. Like the two preceding remedies, this one is miraculous. Even today, after so many years of scientific rationalism, its phenomenal efficiency unquestionably outclasses the most modern discoveries of chemistry.

Luesinum is the last of the three important predispositions that this one man's genius was able to identify. More than a century was to pass before medicine acquired a fourth of equal importance. Medical progress can't be forced. It generally comes from the rare conjunction of an overwhelming calamity and the wisdom of an exceptional person. The most fearful scourge of the beginning of this century is well known to everyone: tuberculosis. The man who most intelligently revealed its workings is known only to homoeopaths. His name is Antoine Nebel, and he deserves immortality for his discovery of the flawed constitution that allows tuberculosis to develop.

TUBERCILINISM

Dr Nebel practised excellent homoeopathy in Lausanne, dying there in 1954 after a long life devoted to his calling. Too involved with his patients the doctor was unable to devote much time to publishing. His offspring, whom I had the honour of caring for, were unable to provide me with any further documentation. There is none. Nebel was quite content to spread the good word like Socrates, and found in a certain Dr Leon Vannier the Plato who was to become the leader of the movement that had begun in Lausanne, and the artisan of a homoeopathic revival in France.

Antoine Nebel had the merit of making homoeopaths understand that tuberculosis was above all a constitutional illness. Admittedly Dr Koch had identified in 1882 the bacteria that leads to tuberculosis and passes for its cause. But this semblance of truth didn't satisfy the Lausanne doctor's curiosity. Using the example of his illustrious precursor's analogical reasoning, he attributed the different morphological signs of tuberculosis to a specific flaw in the constitution which he called 'tuberculinism'. And just like Hering who had analogically found an elegant means to correct the first three constitutions, Nebel countered this tuberculinism that he had invented with the Tuberculinum nosode.

Unlike the other three major biotherapeutics, Tuberculinum is a real nosode since it is prepared directly from a culture of Koch's bacillus. It was the Belgian homeopath Mersch who created it in 1894 and introduced it into the homoeopathic pharmacopoeia. Nebel tried it experimentally at the beginning of this century, giving it a first 'portrait' in 1902. Since then the therapeutic success of Tuberculinum has never ceased to be confirmed. Like the other three biotherapeutics, this unlikely remedy cures. Specific modern antibiotics have not taken its place since it alone is capable of realizing what chemistry is never able to obtain: the elimination of all relapse.

Ever since Mersch, homoeopaths have rounded out their antitubercular panoply with other specific nosodes prepared from other virulent sources and using different techniques. All these remedies have their uses and guarantee homoeopathy a diagnostic and therapeutic finesse that allopaths can't even imagine. I will continue, however, to use the generic term

Tuberculinum to avoid encumbering my text, but will briefly refer to these other nosodes from the same family a little later.

Psora, sycosis, luetism and tuberculinism: these are the four major predispositions recognized by homoeopathy. No others have been discovered. Personally I don't think that there are any others deserving of a place in such illustrious company. Further discoveries can only concern subgroups, types of subsoil that threaten the stability of the four great wavering pillars and the transition of the mysterious forces that link them one to another. I will try to make this clearer by exploring my beliefs more thoroughly later on.

The quadruple setting of Real Medicine is now in place. The four main actors that you will see moving on this stage are the four major constitutional remedies. With Psorinum, Medorrhinum, Luesinum and Tuberculinum the doctor has the fantastic power to regulate, for better or for worse, the primary controlling diagram of vital energy: the genetic code.

NINETEEN

Physiognomy of the four constitutions

All contemporary homoeopaths attribute capital importance to the four major predispositions. Schools of this medical discipline throughout the world devote a substantial part of their programmes to the study of these four fundamental facts of our genetic patrimony. You can well imagine that there is a good reason for this.

Unlike the trivial assaults of chemotherapy, homoeopathic treatment seeks a very particular kind of battle: total war. It strives to reach the evil at its roots in order to destroy it. The battle necessarily takes place at two levels: the front line and the rear lines.

In the first line of battle the ideal remedy is the simillimum. Properly adjusted, the adequate potency is usually enough to re-establish the troubled energetic balance. This is the habitual case with acute illnesses for which the 20 or 30 remedies in your home medicine chest are perfect provided that sequential therapy has already freed the vital energy from its spatiotemporal yoke. But homoeopathy has other ambitions, which go beyond the simple regulation of small acute imbalances. For many of those cases allopathy is almost as effective.

But with chronic illness we come up against another story. Here we are faced with a war of position, static and devious, even if the suddenness of the successive assaults gives the impression of occasional skirmishes. Timely defensive action is no longer sufficient. With each change in the tactical situation, the doctor has to change the similimum or dispense another chemical blow. The therapeutic act must be constantly repeated. But while an allopath has no resource other than the continual repetition of his palliative intervention, a good homoeopath can do much more: he can aim beyond the immediate target at the rear lines as well.

The homoeopath's target is the imbalanced vital energy. But the very nature of this disharmony is not the result of chance. For each patient it is conditioned by the most glaring weakness of their constituent genetic structure. Since the person is made up of four constitutions, it is necessarily the weakness of one of them that gives the tone to the disharmony.

This is why it is essential for the doctor to determine with great precision which of the four constitutions is the least stable. Sometimes there are two or three constitutions showing signs of weakness. In principle the worst one becomes suspect number one and dictates the overall approach to the morbid offensive. If the constitution is discovered quickly, the treatment can be easily adjusted. For every constitutional flaw, homoeopathy can align an entire range of remedies in addition to the four great biotherapeutics mentioned above. This is its most unique feature. By the intrinsic quality of its own vibrations, the immaterial simillimum is necessarily related to the fundamental vibration of one or other of these four dominant predispositions, which in some respects constitute the quadruple archetype of all morbid possibilities.

Hahnemann had already developed a small arsenal of psoric, sycotic and luetic remedies to which Nebel's students added the tuberculinic list. Over the years the homoeopathic Materia Medica has been enriched by many new 'portraits', each with its own qualities, and with which homoeopaths have identified more or less easily with one of the four underlying predispositions.

In order to reach the target and the rear lines simultaneously, the homoeopath must choose the most effective similimum: the one that will both erase the energetic imbalance of the moment and slightly diminish the constitutional instability, which is the hidden reason for the problem. For example, by giving a psoric remedy to a patient who is strongly marked by a psoric heredity, the therapist's work is doubly beneficial since it is correcting the immediate problem and to a lesser extent the flawed tendency which has modelled the present problem. This is true for all morbid states. The doctor is always better placed if he chooses a simillimum from whichever of the four categories of remedies corresponds to the patient's weakest constitution.

If the heredity is in very bad shape owing to simultaneous

weakening of several constitutions, the best similimum will be one taken from the remedies referred to as 'polychrests'. This awkward term was formed from two Greek roots, which imply the multiplicity of services delivered; the polychrest is a remedy that vibrates on several levels at the same time like a musical chord, borrowing its wavelengths from the two or three constitutions to which it belongs.

In the war of attrition that a real doctor wages against chronic illness, the repeated use of appropriate immaterial methods always leads to a very real improvement of the patient's general condition, if not to his complete recovery. This fact cannot be denied, but objectivity forces me to admit that this is where traditional homoeopathy reaches its limits. I have seen too many patients who have been treated for 20 or 30 years by conscientious professionals who follow the Kentist school and who have profoundly suffered from the chronic nature of their condition despite judicious and repeated use of an appropriate simillimum. A traditionalist homoeopath can prescribe correct doses of Pulsatilla to a patient of the Pulsatilla type and he will certainly improve the quality of the patient's life, but he cannot hope to fortify the tubercular constitution, which has determined the patient's propensity to react in the Pulsatilla mode.

Homoeopaths less attached to tradition quickly discovered that the most radical way to make the constitution totally healthy was to have the courage to use the major biotherapeutics themselves. In this the four great remedies are irreplaceable. This is particularly evident when the illness to be treated is directly related to the constitution, that is its instigator. I told a small lie in the preceding chapter in order to lighten my text when I seemed to minimize the role of the mange, gonorrhoea and syphilis. I will now rectify this intentional error by declaring outright that it is impossible to cure these three illnesses definitively, as well as tuberculosis, without the help of the corresponding major biotherapeutic. Allopaths can laugh as much as they wish, convinced that they control the causes with chemotherapy, but their imperfect art will be unable to protect their patients from relapse.

In other chronic illnesses a properly conducted homoeopathic treatment must necessarily also succeed in radically curing the flawed constitution that has allowed the illness to take hold. If the doctor is satisfied with prescribing the similimum of the moment, even if it is perfectly chosen (with or without a computer), he is merely taking care of instead of definitively curing the patient. By not understanding this fairly simple truth, the great majority of contemporary homoeopaths still fail too often in the every bit as simple cure of many repeated illnesses. They say that they are strict Kentists or Hahnemannians and respect the Law of Similarity to the letter, but they have not grasped its essence. They deceive their patients by proposing a lifetime of the remedies that are suggested by Kent's repertory, while one high potency of an appropriate major biotherapeutic would be enough to erase the weighty predisposition that the patient has inherited. Hahnemann wouldn't have hesitated to use these prodigious weapons if they had been at his disposal, since they represent the final accomplishment of his creative thought process brought to fruition by Hering and Nebel. As soon as it is identified, a hereditary pathological tendency must necessarily be corrected. At the very least the doctor must endeavour to halt this implacable method of transmission.

Yes, it is really heredity that we are talking about. If the patient has been giving tuberculinic or sycotic reactional signs for the last 20 years, it is obviously because he has no other way to express himself. And why is this so? Because the biophysical reactions of each living creature are imperatively directed by an intransigent ballet teacher: the genetic code.

In the preceding chapter we saw how the great homoeopathic tradition provides the genetic code with four means of pathological expression as dictated by the four major presdispositions. Our genetic code can't give rise to any other major reactional manifestations. They are quite simply four in number and that's that. It has been thus since the beginning of time, whether the faculty agrees or not.

For the moment only homoeopaths recognize this glaring truth. They search every day, each in their own way, for the symptoms in their patients that will lead to one predisposition or another. The most skilful succeed quickly – in general at first glance – with this essential diagnosis. Less-gifted doctors must resort to the long lists of silly questions extolled by the smaller masters of this art who even call in computers to help. But the speed and methods used to reach this first level of knowledge are not really important. Most important is the investigation itself, which will spare the patient a long and fruitless wait in the shadowy antechamber of traditional homoeopathy when it is possible to open the main door to health with one vigorous push.

To enable curious readers to recognize for themselves the characteristics of their own genetic baggage, I will briefly describe the most visible clues that, once unearthed, clearly point to an underlying constitutional weakness. This short description is not exhaustive but it does present a fairly accurate picture of the general aspects of the four major predispositions.

PSORA

A psoric heredity can be seen primarily in the way the skin looks. It never has the freshness or firmness that are appropriate to youth. The psoric always looks dirty or inadequately washed and can suffer terribly from this air of neglect if he is attentive to appearance and making a good impression. Unfortunately, he can wash ten times a day but the skin will remain as obstinately lack-lustre as his spirits, and in addition it has a bad odour.

It is therefore not surprising that the psoric isn't very cheerful. Essentially pessimistic by nature, he tends to be withdrawn and something of a homebody, disliking travel and social contact. The problems with which he is afflicted show very little tendency towards spontaneous remission. If our patient coughs, he will cough all his life; his migraine headaches and pimples will obstinately refuse treatment. In addition, psorics are always chilly and cannot be warmed up by any heating system. Worse, when the warmth of his home finally removes the uncomfortable impression of being cold 'in the bones', the concentration of positive ions in the atmosphere is usually such that the psoric has to go out for fresh air. This sensitivity to ionic concentrations is characteristic, and the psoric is at his worst when he returns to the plains after a stay in the mountains.

SYCOSIS

A true sycotic is not much better off. At first glance he seems more dynamic than a psoric, but this additional vitality often expresses itself in uncontrolled aggression. This detestable tendency can even be found in the sycotic's sex appeal (this is a trait that he doesn't lack) and can ruin the quality of his relationships with other people. He often deprives himself of the most agreeable pleasures of life by doing everything hastily and at the wrong moment. He is annoying because he is constantly late. In addition he is systematically critical and subject to terrible fits of temper.

The sycotic suffers less from the skin than the psoric, but his mucous discharge is every bit as entrenched, unpleasant and bad smelling as the psoric's eczema or psoriasis. His weak spots are the urogenital system, the tendons and the joints.

He is less sensitive to variations in atmospheric pressure, but dislikes the mountains where his chronic illnesses ruin vacations by their sudden appearance. He feels much better at the seashore, preferring the amenities of a maritime climate to inland dryness. The sycotic is very intolerant of vaccinations, which cause rapid energetic destabilization, a little recognized but essential factor in cancerization.

One last characteristic should be noted. Of the four personalities being caricatured here, the sycotic is the only one who willingly sleeps on his stomach.

LUETISM

The luetic is more appealing than the first two human specimens since he has the major advantage of an impeccable appearance: clean like a newly minted coin and always looking like he has just been unwrapped. Perfectly dressed, he won't tolerate a single spot on his clothing and is obsessed with cleanliness in general. But don't be deceived by this pleasant appearance. Often he tells lies as easily as he breathes and he loves gambling. If honest, he can become a clever businessman but, if his cleverness dominates his code of honour, the luetic won't take long to move into murkier waters.

More inclined to religious domination than to open philosophical reflection, the luetic easily succumbs to fanatic doctrines and can often be trapped by the propaganda of sects. Given to bluffing, he is easily dominated by fashion or an ideology.

The luetic is the typical example of a defective heredity. His flaws are physical as well as moral. Organic deformities are not rare, particularly of the heart and bones. Skeletal pain is frequent and particularly worsened at night. The teeth are poorly implanted and rapidly have cavities despite the best dental hygiene. The luetic child is a born comedian, loving disguises and always clowning around. He is more than active, he's frankly unbearable! This little terror is only calmed down by the periodic high fevers that accompany his frequent swollen throats and earaches.

With age, this hereditary syphilitic will always be attracted by the beauty of the devil, sectarianism, luxury, gambling dens, palaces and the mountains.

TUBERCULINISM

If you think you'll find a more agreeable companion with the tuberculinic, you'll be rapidly disappointed. This timid or extroverted scrawny person is harder to live with than he initially appears owing to his constantly changing moods: overwhelmingly enthusiastic at the beginning of a project he sinks into the deepest apathy at the smallest problem. He can either be something of a Bohemian and disorderly like certain artists, or meticulous and nitpicking instead like some maniac artisan trying to build a masterpiece out of a hundred thousand matches.

His weak point is obviously the respiratory system. Constantly coughing and spitting, he is sensitive to the slightest draught and absolutely intolerant of damp and cold climates. Conscious even before his doctor that his bronchial problems are related to digestion, the tuberculinic is constantly attentive to his digestive tract and worries at the slightest disorder. If he becomes constipated he is lost and he knows it. Loath to make physical or intellectual efforts, he often complains of headaches. The slightest effort causes him to perspire (which he hates).

Overall he is extremely preoccupied with himself and even seems something of a coward. The tuberculinic is afraid of dogs and storms and is as certain as the psoric that he will never recover. His life doesn't really seem worth living, particularly if he is confined by illness or discomfort to a relative immobility. He needs movement at all costs and comes to life if the occasion arises to take a trip.

* * *

These four brief and caricatural portraits each designate the human archetype that the genetic code would produce if it was totally dominated by just one of the major predispositional weaknesses. Obviously such a perverse influence couldn't exist in nature. Only naive homoeopaths could believe that the subtle rules of the game of life could be systematized in this way. You will shortly be able to grasp the extent of their most common and monumental mistake.

TWENTY

Universality of the four predispositions

Homoeopathy has a tremendous advantage over allopathy because through its recognition of the constitutional predispositions it can know the patient's reactional modes to morbid aggression. This fortunate quality is often enhanced by the near-divinatory nature of the diagnosis, which can surprise an uninformed observer. But this forecasting is really quite ordinary. A good homoeopath simply does not allow himself to be surprised. He knows that a given psoric child has a tendency towards a given psoric affliction, that a given tuberculinic or sycotic runs a low risk of luetic complications, favouring instead the ordinary pulmonary or urinary congestion dictated by that dual constitutional weakness.

This enormous superiority in forecasting does have one major disadvantage. It can lead to preconceived ideas, those small sins of the intellectual and the fatal pillow of laziness to the strategist. If too efficient at labelling, a methodical mind can end up seeing nothing but the labels, forgetting that all ordering is merely a convention and one that requires revision when the viewpoint changes. Life itself is nothing but change, undergoing the pitiless sovereignty of our old friend time. We think and act differently in youth and in maturity, our illnesses aren't the same, and our reactions change over the years.

I am not putting forward these commonplace remarks to play the philosopher, but rather to draw your attention to what is essentially artificial in the four descriptions presented in the last chapter. By following them too blindly, the doctor risks fixing his assessment in a restricted approach that is very detrimental to the patient. This short-cut can lead to the fatal impasse where homoeopathy often gets lost, the classic trap whose dangers I will here denounce.

From the first moment of initiation the neophyte is tempted to try the amusing parlour game of classifying family and friends into one of the main categories. The tendency is even stronger if their teachers delight in talking about their difficult 'tuberculinic' cases, nice little 'psorics' and amusing 'luetics'. But not all students are taken in.

My wife, who combines a lively critical mind with healthy common sense, often accompanied me to the classes organized by my teacher. She listened attentively to the lessons and with amusement to our subsequent debates. Her sound judgement was never tainted by a preference for one school or another. One day she finally pronounced sentence on our proceedings: 'Everyone can recognize themselves in every one of the portraits! Everyone has tended to be chilly at some time in their life, has been afraid of big dogs, of storms or of the future. Any child benefits from a stay in the mountains or by the sea. And who would be crazy enough to prefer misery to riches and cleanliness? And who doesn't like to travel? And who has never at one point or another slept happily on their stomach?' To her these rules of classification seemed both imprecise and ridiculous. The classifications themselves became futile and derisory.

After thinking about her arguments I was obliged to agree with her up to a certain point. You yourselves have also certainly noticed that we all present most of the signs and symptoms mentioned above at one point or another in our lives. As for me, I admit to having been susceptible to cold as a child, having no fear of storms, but hating unplanned events. Now I'm always warm, I'm afraid of thunder and I love change. I slept for years on my stomach and now I go to sleep on my back. I'm a real homebody, but I love to travel. Each of us can probably come up with a similar list of obvious contradictions that demolish the simplistic theory. This could only mean one of two things. Either the homoeopaths are wrong and their predispositional system a trap or the classification is meaningful but only under certain conditions.

Since then I have too often been able to verify the accuracy of the predispositional system to deny its value. The theory is correct, provided that our old friend time is right there in the middle. Yes, this is a constant of the sciences of life. We always find this saturnine concept at the centre of any energetic phenomenon that is spatiotemporal by definition. Theorists should never forget this. Most homoeopaths unfortunately forget that life is change and make the mistake of staying for good with the first label given to their patients. If a patient is 'sycotic', he will be treated as 'sycotic' for 20 years. If another one is deemed 'tuberculinic', he will be treated as such for life. This classic error is even more unfortunate since it is based on a simple flaw of reasoning. As a result of all their analogical thinking homoeopaths often lose their sense of logic. Logic is childlike and nourished by the obvious.

It is obvious that, with a little goodwill, the doctor can find a nice group of symptoms for each of the four predispositions in any patient's anamnesis. But why aren't these signs permanent if they are representative of the underlying constitution? Isn't the constitution a fundamental given by definition? How can a doctor declare a patient 'luetic' when his past is full of psoric, tuberculinic and sycotic clues? If the signs that reveal the other predispositions aren't apparent at the time of diagnosis, then there is only one logical explanation the doctor can give to this anomaly: at the time of diagnosis, the dominant signs momentarily eclipse the others. This doesn't authorize the homoeopath to forget those that are seemingly absent. What would you think of an archaeologist who denied the Romanesque origins of a building simply because a later builder had embellished it with Gothic arches?

I did not wish to make the same mistake by accepting uncritically the imperfect teachings of the homoeopaths. I am of too saturnine a temperament to neglect the shadowy god who holds out the hour-glass and the scythe. Beginning in 1976, I systematically considered that the genetic baggage of each of my patients included all four fundamental threats that rule over the individual destabilization of vital energy. One after the other they imprint and distort in their own way the wonderful space–time cluster that structures living matter. This work of profound structuring does not pass unnoticed on the surface. It gives a particular style to all the vital reactions analysed by the doctor, thereby creating in each patient a composite mask overlaying the true face of the principal predisposition.

If one of the four constitutions seems to eclipse the others at the time of diagnosis, the observer must not conclude that the rival genetic instructions have been definitively lost or cancelled. The information in a computer programme is not erased when the user changes programmes. Our genetic code is nothing more than a fabulous computer memory. It contains all the information necessary to life, but makes it available only wisely and at the right time. By minutely studying the anamneses of my patients I realized that they had all been subjected to the structural rules of the four archetypes at one moment or another in their lives. I rapidly acquired the conviction that **every one of us has been in turn psoric, tuberculinic, sycotic and luetic**.

What should be the attitude of a homoeopath who is aware of the strength of his weapons? He knows that the correctly chosen simillimum can reach both the front and the rear lines. He knows how to complement this tactical action with the strategic effect of a major biotherapeutic for the constitution (that long–range missile bringing help to the weakened defence of a destabilized base from which the morbid attack started). Logically there is no reason for the doctor to deprive the other defensive systems of the fantastic energetic support that the key constitutional nosodes bring so rapidly to their respective goals. Why not stimulate them as well? The act is so simple! All it requires is to prescribe to each patient a fairly high potency of each of the four great remedies.

The surprising results confirm this hypothesis to be correct. Starting in 1976 I systematically – in complete contradiction with official homoeopathic doctrine – bestowed a quadruple biotherapeutic barrage on each of my patients. Naturally I had first reinstated the best energetic balance I could through the methodical and meticulous application of my sequential isotherapy. I was already aware of the fact that, in working on the four major constitutions, I was touching the most intimate mechanisms of genetic regulation. I had always thought it stupid and dangerous to try to correct a prenatal energetic conflict (this is precisely what we are talking about) before having first unknotted the spatiotemporal imbroglio of the patient's life. Hering's Law is valid for any chronology, and the Mikado effect relentlessly penalizes those who imprudently ignore it.

In fact I have to point out here that I am amazed to see how carelessly the most reputed homoeopaths use the major constitutional remedies, sometimes even at the beginning of a treatment or starting at the second or third visit. This folly is even more dangerous when certain colleagues in a hurry don't hesitate to prescribe very high potencies – 50,000 or 100,000K (written LM or CM in Latin) – without knowing the elementary principles of prior cleansing with the nosodes. I strongly advise any patient who receives one of the four biotherapeutics to ask their doctor if he has first eliminated all the accumulated astral stickiness of their lives. If the answer is negative, or worse if the doctor doesn't know what you're talking about, you are better off interrupting your treatment and waiting until the homoeopath has read this book! On the other hand, if the principal destabilizing events have been noted and correctly neutralized by a good isosequential therapy, then use of the four great remedies brings about a wonderful improvement in health for the chronically ill patient who receives them.

To convince you, here are the plain facts as I have observed them daily in my office over the years. Since they are an obvious contradiction of traditional homoeopathic doctrine, and since no theory has ever been able to refute the direct facts of reality, I think that this doctrine must be urgently modified.

Starting in 1976, I gave all my patients Psorinum up to the XMK potency whether they were psoric or not after having properly healed their past of the various wounds inflicted by life. In patients with a strong psoric heredity I naturally observed the usual reactions, which any homoeopath would expect following administration of such a remedy: all kinds of increased skin eliminations, violent itching, rashes and alarming swelling. The eczema and psoriasis that had been pushed 'inside' by the dermatologists' cortisone ointments rediscovered their natural tendency – unfortunate, but beneficial – to move towards the outside. The asthmas, croups and other bronchial ailments appeared in all their glory, accomplishing the classic homoeopathic aggravation of morbid symptoms then subsequently rapidly diminishing or disappearing. This is normal in homoeopathy. First there is always a momentary awakening of the ailment before the beneficial corrective effect of the proper remedy can occur.

For each of my psoric patients I witnessed this increase of dermatological, respiratory, digestive or neurological problems and, once the storm had passed, I had the intense joy of seeing them rapidly improve – much more rapidly than if I had obeyed the fixed orthodoxy of the classical homoeopaths. But this fairly commonplace pleasure, which is known to other biotherapeutic strategists, can't even be compared to the heady intoxication that

I felt upon realizing what was taking place with my other, non-psoric patients.

All the tuberculinics, sycotics and luetics who had also received Psorinum were manifesting the same psoric symptoms as the psorics! Now here was something that didn't correspond at all to the theory of my learned teachers. But I wasn't dreaming. The same dermatological, bronchial and neurological aggravations appeared in my consulting rooms. The complaints were clearly not as serious, but the morbid signs were nevertheless very real and unquestionably 'psoric'.

Turning my back on dogma, I logically concluded that psora must be universal and that Psorinum was necessary to anyone who wanted to achieve the astonishing sense of well-being of recovered energetic balance. I had exactly the same experience when I administered Tuberculinum, Medorrhinum and Luesinum to all my patients. In every single one of them I set in motion the same reactional signs, more or less violent and beneficial, depending on the level of health of the underlying constitution.

Hahnemann himself had already sensed the universality of psora, to which he devoted a significant part of his treatise on chronic illness. He didn't live long enough to experiment with Psorinum, the perfect remedy that Hering had potentized in 1834, 9 years before his death. The master who had, without knowing it, discovered the first of the four plans of our genetic code never realized how close he had been to the truth. With sycosis and luetism, which he stigmatized with talent, Hahnemann seems not to have followed his intuition with the same degree of success as he failed to attribute the same universality to these two predispositions. He was never to know their biotherapeutics either. As for tuberculinism, it had to wait until Nebel, who hit upon the concept following Koch's discovery of his bacteria.

The era of pioneers is behind us. The four great predispositions and their four great regulators are now known to all homoeopaths. Their respective importance is, however, far from being unanimously recognized by all my colleagues. Most still insist on giving their patients one label or another although **we all have our origins in the same four constitutions**. Most doctors are not aware that these four constitutions are really just the reactional expressions of the four directing impulses of our common and equal genetic codes.

Are they really all the same? The answer is an emphatic **yes**, with one small precision, modest and yet essential, which is the golden key of Real Medicine.

TWENTY-ONE

The Law of the Succession of Forces

We have finally reached the heart of our theoretical and practical study of the bioenergetic phenomenon that is usually called 'life'. I will now ask the reader to excuse my presumption in requiring him to abandon momentarily the intellectual habits of logical reasoning and borrow from his intuition the analogical method of the propagation of ideas. I can think of no other way that will enable him to stay with me throughout this chapter on the fabulous cosmic merry-go-round, which governs the slow humanizing materialization of the primordial life spark. He will thus grasp, much more quickly, the irresistible symbolism of the number four, and the numerological inspiration of these lines and of Real Medicine.

Four predispositions, four remedies, four seasons, four forces: there will be nothing but this rhythm of four in the following pages. This obsessive tetralogy took hold of my right brain one day and wouldn't leave me in peace until the execution of the present work.

It all started with the contradictory shock arising from the observation of facts. The close study of anamneses had shown me that we are all fashioned by the four predispositions. My wife was right, and the dogmatists wrong. Feminine intuition in fact always grasps a biological reality better than the canniest of reasoning.

Since this quadruple label was immediately bestowed on all my patients, I logically had to help all of them by giving everyone the four great remedies. But how to go about doing this? I couldn't just fire away immediately with all my heavy artillery! The four great biotherapeutics can't be used simultaneously without risk of chaos in the field. They have to be prescribed one after the other. But what to do?

Essential questions had to be answered. Which one should begin? Is it the same for everyone? Was there a predetermined order for the other three? Once again it was direct observation of the real world and simple common sense that pointed me in the right direction.

Beginning at the end of 1976, I had succeeded in an atmosphere of enthusiasm in converting to homoeopathy my first chronically ill patients, thrilled at discovering a new hope of recovery through this change in strategy. I had freed them from their successive immaterial shackles through the rigorously chronological sequential therapy based on the shaky data of the Vollian approach.

Having brought them to this stage of 'cleanliness' by my energetic cleaning process, I was pleased to see that they had all recovered an excellent Yin–Yang balance at the 12 terminal or starting points of the meridians tested with Voll's method. I will explain later the importance of this observation. Logically I was in a position to pronounce them cured since health is defined precisely by the recovery of energetic balance. And, to tell the truth, they were all effectively vastly improved in their general condition. The innumerable small problems that were noted throughout the cure had all disappeared as if by magic. Gone were the constant colds, chronic coughs, indigestion and other functional problems. And there was an additional invaluable benefit. Their defensive ability to ward off new morbid attacks now seemed activated. Overall, my patients seemed for the most part to have recovered their ability to react to new energetic aggressions with appropriate corrective measures.

Yet the principal signs of the chronic ailments still showed an unfortunate tendency to reappear in the forefront as soon as favourable conditions for a relapse appeared: excessive food, atmospheric change, dust, pollen or other irritants, for example. My chronic cases were therefore not cured despite the apparent stability of their general energetic equilibrium as certified by my ohmmetric readings.

At this stage of the treatment a good experienced homoeopath or acupuncturist should know that a definitive recovery can be obtained only by balancing the inherited impulses, those 'ancestral energies' described by the Chinese. In fact it is a stabilization of the constitution that is necessary, a purging of the genetic code to remove the energetic distortions received before birth or conception. I know that it isn't easy to correct this problem with acupuncture; hundreds of people have tried for many years. But in homoeopathy I think the feat is possible. This is how it is done.

In the preceding chapter you saw how I reached the conviction that all of our genetic codes carry the same four great weaknesses. You also know how I claim to correct this handicap. As for the question of which biotherapeutic should be given first, the answer is now clear and unequivocal: Psorinum must always be given first.

With each of my patients who reached this initial stage of cleanliness at the end of the corrective sequence I noticed that it was curiously and unquestionably always psora that was the first of the predispositions to show itself. With patients who were psoric this was obvious, but if the patient happened to have come to see me for a typically luetic complaint, he found himself at this stage of my preliminary treatment manifesting typically psoric symptoms along with his usual luetic nature. This curiosity repeated itself with all my patients at this stage of the treatment independently of their predispositional signs. I logically concluded that not only was psora universal, but that it was also the most readily disposed to unveil itself. It leapt to the surface as soon as it was called, like a jack-in-the-box when you take off the cover.

The uniform persistence of resurgent psoric symptoms can't escape an attentive observer. Even if the other predispositional signs seemed to dominate the clinical picture, I found that the constant presence of two or three psoric symptoms required the prescribing of the first major biotherapeutic. This primacy of psora in the hierarchy of structural forces didn't escape Hahnemann. Today it appears even more forcefully when homoeopaths during their treatments use certain remedies that are designed to strengthen the constitution. I have intentionally not mentioned them to avoid turning my book into a treatise. All you need know is that these remedies complete the recovery of a patient who has a sound genetic patrimony, but give rise to certain superficial reactions in those less well endowed. These reactions are generally quite clearly psoric in nature.

To remove my remaining hesitations at invariably prescribing Psorinum first, I used experimentally a particular technique of radiesthesia invented for this purpose, which involves the comparative sensibility of the key meridian. As these experiments also convinced me of the constant and total 'chronological' primacy of psora over the other diatheses, I irrevocably decided in 1976 to begin all my subsequent constitutional treatments with Psorinum. I have invariably respected this discipline for the past 8 years. For each patient who reaches the end of the isosequential cleansing I start the predispositional phase of my intervention in an identical manner by prescribing progressively stronger potencies of Psorinum. I find it necessary to give this first biotherapeutic in a high potency. After some experimenting I found that 10,000K seems to be the most useful, and I never go beyond this threshold at the outset.

Naturally, if the patient shows psoric signs right away that are very characteristic of the major related remedies, I then prescribe these remedies immediately since I consider them to be 'inductors' of psora. I therefore often give Sulphur, Antimonium crudum or Arsenicum album to prepare the way for the great biotherapeutic. But I must always, yes always, conclude this approach phase with Psorinum, even if the patient is jovial, flushed and obese! Traditional Hahnemannian or Kentist homoeopaths can raise their hands to the heavens and cry scandal if they so wish, but I stand my ground. Psorinum simply cannot be replaced in any effort to regulate the genetic code, and must always be given first. **Its impact on superior space–time awakens the first of the four great forces by its resonance**.

* * *

Let us pause for a moment at this cryptic statement and pursue the investigation in a scientific way by verifying the effects of this treatment on the patients. Plenty of examples exist. I've often had to laugh at the naivety of the authors of certain scholarly articles who claim to draw conclusions of universal meaning based on the statistical study of small series of 20 or 30 cases. Though still modest, my experience is considerably greater. I have administered Psorinum over 3,000 times and have been able to verify unequivocally the therapeutic effects of this approach.

As I mentioned earlier, in all markedly psoric patients the momentary worsening of the morbid symptomatology was obvious. The preceding chapter also indicated that the same psoric symptoms appeared in all the other diatheses. What you don't know yet is what became of these 3,000 chronically ill patients with whom I began this genetic 'cleansing' in such a cavalier manner. The unfolding of an illness following the doctor's intervention is called a 'catamnesis'. It is every bit as instructive as an anamnesis when it comes to establishing the main lines of a new medical philosophy.

What the catamnesis revealed was quite simply the answer to the questions I raised at the beginning of this chapter. After Psorinum the other three biotherapeutics must also be given **to all patients and in a specific order**.

But before unveiling the absolute simplicity of the 'Law of the Succession of Forces', which is the ultimate outcome of my sequential therapy, I must first briefly outline the quintessence of the observations that led to its discovery.

The administration of Psorinum starts a surface agitation, which can lead to a symptomatic crisis. To diminish slightly the disagreeable side of this foreseeable reaction it is very helpful to prescribe 'draining' remedies. In some respects they act as counterparts of the inductors mentioned earlier by also helping the shock wave to pass. A rough comparison would be a humpback structure facilitating the passage over a large pipe temporarily laid across a roadway.

However, the 'drainer' should not be prescribed in too high a potency, to avoid interference with the Psorinum vibrations. To avoid this risk I use certain commercial preparations that, heretically, mix a number of proven remedies in very low potencies. This is perfectly contrary to Hahnemann's teaching, which requires seeking the precise simillimum, but it is nevertheless efficient and it is certainly very gentle. But to help Psorinum's subtle action even better, I am generally content with the regulatory effects of correctly activated oligoelements (*see* Glossary). I have been using these catalysts daily for the last 15 years instead of homoeopathic 'drainers' and have never been disappointed. They admirably complement the deep and violent activity of the biotherapeutic with their gentle effects. It was Dr Ménétrier who first noticed that the psoric predisposition could be corrected with manganese (Mn). He also described the slow transformation of this primitive predisposition into a tubercular constitution over time. The ideal stabilizer of this second weakness is no longer manganese alone, but manganese supplemented by copper (Cu). By giving Mn then Mn–Cu to his patient, an unsuspecting therapist exactly reproduces what nature does 'spontaneously' under the orders of Psorinum by itself.

We are now approaching the inner workings of the succession of forces. After administration of the great remedy, the clinical picture is dominated by symptoms of the 'drainers'. These then diminish and become the symptoms brought out by the inductors of the next predisposition. The next predisposition takes over, must in turn be stabilized by other 'drainers', which are transformed into inductors of the next predisposition, and so on and so forth.This is the exact description of the adventure of my 3,000 psorics 'cleansed' by Psorinum. In the weeks following administration of the great remedy they all showed varying degrees of clinical signs warranting psoric 'draining'. They then over time all showed symptoms indicating the induction of the next predisposition. Without exception this new predisposition took the shape of tuberculinism, in perfect agreement with the previsional theory of Ménétrier's biological catalysis.

What was my reaction? After a new radiesthesic verification I unhesitatingly administered Tuberculinum and **restarted, by resonance, the second of the four great forces**.

* * *

To help you grasp the heretical nature of this method, which is so contrary to the individualist aspirations of the homoeopathic school, I will present the following archiclassical example of a young luetic patient brought to me in desperation by his parents who had exhausted the limited means of allopathy. The 4- or 5-year-old boy before me behaved in a clownish and grimacing manner as soon as he set foot in my consulting room, as well as displaying an exasperating level of energy. He climbed all over the furniture, touched everything in sight, refused to sit still and was, in short, unbearable. Ever since his first vaccinations this little mercurian's health had vanished in a succession of earaches, sore throats, bronchitis and colds. His short life had been spent between the waiting rooms of the paediatrician and the ENT specialist. The former, responsible for the energetic destabilization, had worsened the situation through chemical intoxication. The latter, every bit as ignorant of the real cause of the problem, had attempted the impossible in trying to prevent the energetic dissipation with the help of costly techniques. Everything had been in vain. Recovery finally started the day the parents understood that the allopathic doctors didn't know their business.

With me the child was first freed from his iatrogenic bonds and other astral stickiness. I then went after the constitution from the angle of psora, contrary to homoeopathic dogma, which would have indicated Luesinum. What was going to happen? Following the reactions of psoric elimination I was expecting a resurgence of the luetic signs. They didn't take long to appear. Was I now supposed to give Luesinum? Logically yes, but once again no. The Law of the Succession of Forces, which I have derived through observation, gives priority to Tuberculinum for all patients irrespective of their illnesses. In the predispositional hierarchy, tuberculinism is always second. I have verified this over 3,000 times with my own eyes, and verify it daily with my radiesthesic techniques. This natural order must be respected.

And which remedy is third? Let us go back to my little luetic patient so that you can follow the cautious approach of an impartial observer. First he received Psorinum, then Tuberculinum. And how had he changed? Obviously his behaviour was modified by the impact of the second great nosode. Like hundreds of other luetic children that I have cured of their chronic ear and throat problems, my patient now had all the symptoms indicative of tuberculinic draining mixed with the luetic signs. This picture was gradually replaced by the inductive signs of the next predisposition. Was it finally going to be luetism? No, once again I had to constrain myself to the biotherapeutic that all my observations as well as the radiesthesic check unanimously imposed: Medorrhinum. In the hierarchical order of succession, sycosis is the third predisposition and its biotherapeutic **awakens, by resonance, the third of the four great forces**.

* * *

Following this energetic blow my little patient showed the various signs of sycotic draining, just like the 3,000 other recipients of this treatment. He was now at last able to give free play to his luetic temperament in the induction of the fourth predispositional manifestation: luetism. There is often at this stage a tremendous increase in the habitual symptoms. The child had his 20th case of otitis and 30th severe throat inflammation, which I was able to cure without difficulty using the oligo-element copper, and the good little 'Conod's drops', a local speciality as efficient as it is heretical. (The unquestionable efficiency of this type of 'pluralist' preparation which mixes several elements sacrilegiously, is striking proof of the invalidity of the rigid 'unicist' doctrine.) To finish my work and bring this beneficial cleansing to a close, I gave the fourth great biotherapeutic: Luesinum. This last essential impulse **shakes, by resonance, the fourth and last of the great forces**. The subsequent luetic draining can create a final mercurian crisis of ENT pathology, which ancient medical astrology and homoeopathy both treat effectively with mercury. Generally, after this dramatic cure, the chronic illness is finished.

* * *

For children of healthy parents with no consanguinity, this first biotherapeutic incursion into the four hidden supports of the genetic code is enough to guarantee an enduring stability of the energetic balance which was first reinstated by sequential isotherapy. I never go beyond a potency of 10,000K for this first quadruple attack which I call the 'EI cycle'. (I will explain in a minute the motive behind the cyclical representation. As for the letter E, I like its four clear lines and graphics, that ideally symbolize the four constituent powers of primitive energy. The fact that it is both the initial of this mathematical concept and my own name can only contribute (unfortunately!) to my inventor's vanity.)

As for moderately destabilized adults, the EI cycle is able to re-establish the solidity of the constitution, that guarantee of subsequent good health. However, the fact is that not all of my 3,000 patients treated in this way recovered. Both the more severely debilitated children and the adults suffering from chronic illnesses needed more than this first modest regulation. But what could be done, what could be given after Luesinum XM? Since the great precursors had not invented any other diatheses I was not about to invent a fifth one myself.

There was only one way out. I had to increase the depth of my work by playing the same diathesic sequence again in another key. Obviously the impact of the XM powers hadn't been enough to obtain the required correction of the deeply tainted genetic instructions. I therefore had to continue with a stronger power after Luesinum XM. But which one? Should I give another high potency of Luesinum? Of course not, since I had already put Luesinum at the last place in the genetic sequence. It seemed simplest to maintain the same order and start the work again at the beginning. This is how the idea of cycles of increased power came to me.

So I followed my first heredosequential intervention with a second incursion into the four predispositions using the same biotherapeutics, but this time potentized to 50,000K (abbreviated as LMK). This is the EII cycle. Like the first one, it is rigorously sequential and doesn't permit of any deviation from the majestic succession of forces: Psorinum, Tuberculinum, Medorrhinum and Luesinum. The mysterious sequence is inalterable.

The EII cycle is extraordinarily efficient. It is extremely rare that a chronic illness resists if the treatment is properly administered in a timely fashion. If the constitution is really too weak, the doctor can try one last time with the EIII cycle, administering the same remedies in the same order but potentized to the 100,000th power (CM). I am personally extremely reticent to try anything more violent and I have never experimented with the EIV or EV cycles which theoretically could exist using powers of 500,000 or 1 million. The reason for this moderation is actually quite simple. The first two cycles are adequate in the immense majority of cases durably to re-establish health.

I must, however, mention one more essential detail. It complements the notion of cycles with the rhythm of the seasons, which play such an important role in all life phenomena. No practical information on this subject exists in any homoeopathic book since neither Hahnemann, Hering nor any of their successors had the intuition to consider the great predispositions as elements of a cycle. Only Nebel would have been in a position to discover this since his precursors were of course not even aware of the fourth great predisposition which he had discovered.

I established the relationship between the two quadralogies by a simple pirouette of analogical reasoning. As long as I was involved only in the EI sequence there was no real reason for me to be concerned about the depth of the activity. Doses of XM are active only for about 6 weeks and the patient's reactions can be monitored from one visit to the next. But the situation is totally different with doses of LM, which as I have said, are really long-range missiles. Two to three months are required by the organism to execute fully the condensed vibrational instructions of an LM dose. The doctor can therefore prescribe each of the four great remedies only once a year.

Once a year, 3 months for each, four in a row, and the year is over. And suddenly it was clear somewhere in my right brain: the four predispositions were the daughters, or at least the cousins, of the four seasons. I immediately verified this intuition by submitting it to the double test of practice and comparative radiesthesic analysis, and I made a surprising discovery: all my chronic patients who had finished the EI sequence and were relatively well stabilized began once again to show signs of psoric instability at the beginning of the autumn. The duration of the period of stability, be it 6 months or 30 days, didn't change a thing. These patients reappeared at my office at the beginning of September. Their weakness seemed even more paradoxical since all of them had received their basic constitutional remedy at the end of the treatment, which was supposed to have fortified them. (I now use these remedies only as indicators of the degree of constitutional stability. If the patient barely reacts on taking them then the constitution is stable. If there are psoric reactions then I know the heredity must be corrected more vigorously.)

It seemed that I wasn't wrong. At least the first predisposition seemed clearly linked to autumn. And the more that I thought about it, the clearer it became that the predispositions, like the seasons, were merely the successive faces of an eternal renewal. We are all dominated by the reactional variations imposed by nature and which the ancient Chinese observed so accurately. In fact we can all perceive this diversity. Who has never been taken with psoric spleen at the onset of autumn, suffered from tuberculinic bronchitis in winter, felt the typically sycotic sexual vitality of spring and the characteristically luetic effects of unexpected sore throats in summer?

If the heredity is sound the health is robust and we remain impervious to the assaults of the seasons. If the heredity is only slightly altered, regulation with the biotherapeutic sequence at doses of XM is enough to re-establish health. This is the case with a majority of slightly chronically ill patients (those with constant allergic colds, repeated bad throats, otitis, etc). Since they don't act over a long time period, the XM doses can be administered outside their respective seasons. Only the sequential order is unalterable: Psorinum – Tuberculinum – Medorrhinum – Luesinum.

Things are completely different when the chronic illness resists the EI cycle. Knowing that I will have to use the LM powers and that each one will 'work' for 3 months, logic requires me to place my interventions at the right moment. Ever since 1977 I have refrained from giving the major biotherapeutics outside their seasons. I still allow myself a certain amount of variation for the EI cycle, but with the second I am rigorously precise. I usually start the EII cycle at the autumn equinox with Psorinum LM, then Tuberculinum LM at the winter solstice, Medorrhinum LM at the spring equinox and Luesinum LM to end the cycle at the summer solstice.

I consider this last detail to be essential. Unfortunately almost all homoeopaths manipulate the high predispositional potencies without any reference to the seasons. The most reputed teachers find it perfectly normal to prescribe Psorinum LM in January and Luesinum LM in November if the Law of Similarities seems to indicate those remedies. I don't agree with this approach. In my opinion the fundamental law of homoeopathy must be applied using both more general and more restrictive criteria as soon as we go beyond the vital disharmony of an individual to that of his archetype, the human being.

Even if they don't realize it, homoeopaths have the power through the four great biotherapeutics to correct the genetic code (they can also deregulate it as well!). It is imperative that doctors realize this immediately since genetic surgery is on the verge of committing science to a road of ultimate madness. It would be so much wiser to correct the imperfections of nature with the means that nature offers. The four great remedies are the wonderful spatio-temporal prolongations of the four major genetic structures. They are the levers by which the doctor can regenerate the tired course of the merry-go-round of the four great forces.

What are these mythical entities which have presented themselves to humanity's consciousness since the beginning of time in the symbolic form of a revolving cross? No one really knows. Contemporary physicists also speak of the four aspects of primal energy, but I never find in their descriptions the wonderful simplicity of the sacred cross of Mu. I do know instinctively that the four great forces animate with the same sovereign authority everything that has taken form in our universe.

The allopaths who may have ventured into these pages will have found them insane. The homoeopaths who are trapped in dogma will feel the same. No matter. In reality, the medicine that is presented here to a large audience is neither medical care nor homoeopathy. It doesn't pay much attention to palliative solutions. It goes straight to the point and claims to be able to heal by central regulation. It is Real Medicine.

TWENTY-TWO

Complete sequential therapy

The confession that I owe everyone seeking help and recovery through my method cannot be put off any longer. The moment of truth has arrived! Since 1977 I have given all my patients, whether men, women or children, the same basic treatment. I have done this irrespective of the illness I was being consulted about, in total contradiction to the commonly held opinion of homoeopaths: the need for an individual and specific medicine. What could appear at first sight to be nothing more than a joke is in fact the unembellished truth.

Why then should I even call myself a homoeopath? Real Medicine isn't homoeopathy any more than it is allopathy. More than anything else it is isopathic and sequential, borrowing only the analogical reasoning and immaterial weapons of the Hahnemannian method.

Obviously, though, the method used to administer the corrective sequence must be rigorously adapted to each patient based on the events that have marked the skein of his life. In this respect my simplistic method achieves a degree of personalization unequalled by any other. Despite the seeming banality of the 20 or 30 causes of disorder that are usually identified, the number of their mathematical combinations is far greater than one might think. But as soon as the first part of the treatment is finished the patient loses all right to an individualization of my rescue efforts!

As soon as we arrive at the constitution, M or Mme Dupont lose their identity and appear in their original simplicity of *Homo sapiens.* Their vital energy is reduced to the ancestral energy contained in the double helix of DNA, or, more specifically in the revolving wheel of the four antagonistic and complementary forces which imposes on our initial structural code, the 'power-form' laid down by the original Law.

Homoeopathic doctrine maintains the flattering idea of a personalized treatment. The individualization of the remedy is of course appropriate as long as the patient has not regained his original energetic purity. But it must disappear in favour of the inalterable genetic sequence as soon as the homoeopath brings into play the formidable power of the four great biotherapeutics. If the doctor is not familiar with the Law of the Succession of Forces and gives the Tuberculinum nosode only to an established tuberculinic, then he is laying down a specific subsequent orientation from which the patient will suffer for the rest of his life. There is even a risk that after 20 years of treatment the patient will become definitively 'individualized' in one of the innumerable tuberculinic roles. The only correct way to fortify a tuberculinic (and the only intelligent medical way to prevent tuberculosis) is to prescribe the four great remedies in the sequential order of the four forces and the four seasons. All other flaws of the constitution are corrected, without exception, in the same way.

Does this method seem too simple, even too simplistic? Is it still possible to speak here of a medical art? I hesitated for a very long time before publishing this therapeutic method, which seems a bit like a steamroller crushing the delicate flower-beds of homoeopathy. It had already taken me a long time to admit the striking evidence of the Law of the Succession of Forces. Was it possible that truth could be so simple? Could such a childlike concept of health one day seem obvious to everyone? After considerable thought it seemed clear to me that the order of precedence of the predispositions wasn't more absurd or less serious than the majestic sequence of the seasons recognized alike by the scientist and the child.

Luckily doctors have a tremendous advantage over other observers of the human condition in their ability to verify immediately their theoretical reasoning. The irrefutable proof of the accuracy of their analyses has a wonderful name: total recovery. This supreme gift of life stops all quarrels and guarantees a deserved prestige to the winning method. Over the years during which I have administered the complete sequential therapy to all my patients I have witnessed the amazing efficiency of the method, provided of course that it was started in time. Like any doctor I have also naturally had many failures, as much due to my own inadequacies as to the usual causes of medical impotence. But I have also encountered so many unhoped-for successes that my remaining doubts have vanished over the years.

And, believe me, a lot of proof was required to convince me in the first place. I would even say that the hardest part for me was to accept my successes. Because of them I had committed the hangable offence of losing my clientele! After 2 or 3 years of complete sequential therapy most of my patients stopped reappearing in my consulting rooms. This is extremely worrying when a doctor has become used to seeing the same faces every 6 or 8 weeks and suddenly the regular contact disappears. Did I miss an important diagnosis? Did I upset the patient in a tactless manner? Had the treatment been a complete failure? Luckily Lausanne is a small city and news gets around very quickly. During the first years I would anxiously ask any ex-patients who I would chance upon in the street whether they had been satisfied with the treatment. 'But of course, doctor! What do you think? Ever since taking your little pills I've felt wonderful. I'm cured. That's why you don't see me at your office any more.'

Phew! that was quite a relief. My doubts disappeared for ever when for every politely evasive reply I could count ten along the lines of 'My son has never been sick again since he took your pills. When I think of all those visits to the paediatrician I blame myself for not having come to see you sooner . . . '

So I wasn't dreaming; the sequential therapy did cure. As a result I had to modify my appointment methods fairly smartly. For years I had enjoyed the vain satisfaction of a 'successful' doctor who could only offer appointments at some vague date in the far future, and then suddenly, like a beginner, I had to accept two or three new cases a day in order to keep my practice going. My situation was made even more delicate by the fact that once my patients were 'back on their feet' they acquired at my instigation their own homoeopathic medicine chests and easily took care of occasional lapses in their restored energetic balances without my help.

Perhaps I am optimistic by nature or tremendously presumptuous. According to my jealous colleagues I am only taking care of healthy people. But why then were they not capable of 'healing' the imaginary sicknesses of these patients they had treated for years with chemicals or homoeopathy before losing their confidence? Need I add that I am rarely the first doctor consulted? The grip of the 'medical business' on our populations is unfortunately still so strong that patients often discover too late the luminous aspect of Real Medicine. Please believe me when I say that some of the cases I mention in this book would have cost society a lot less and would have been cured a lot more quickly if the patients had encountered immaterial techniques a little earlier. I can say the same about hundreds of other 'hypochondriacs' who honoured me with their trust.

Is it then a question of luck? I have already told you what I think of spontaneous remissions. I would really be blessed by the gods if chronic illnesses became child's play as soon as they walked through my consulting rooms door. No, the definitive proof of the validity of an experiment lies in being able to reproduce its results. Let us therefore look at what the method alone does when the practitioner changes.

In 1979 I took care of a young woman who very obviously had a real interest in the world of medicine. This patient – who wishes to remain anonymous – interrupted her medical studies when she married but continued to follow the courses as an unregistered student. Frustrated by the one-sidedness of official teaching, she had rapidly become interested in less materialistic therapies and had followed courses at the two homoeopathic schools that had recently opened in Lausanne. She compared these Hahnemannian and Vollian methods with mine during the treatment I prescribed and afterwards during the short apprenticeship that she did in my consulting rooms the following year. Completely seduced by the logical simplicity of the complete sequential therapy, she rapidly became an enthusiastic follower. Shortly thereafter she opened a naturopathic practice and now treats patients similar to mine who have been disappointed by chemotherapeutic medicine.

Is she satisfied with her practice? I think I can say yes, given that her successes are as enviable as my own. Please don't think that the cases handled by this therapist with no diploma are any easier than the ones mentioned in these pages. Most of the chronic illnesses she has cured were diagnosed and unsuccessfully treated at length by our most reputed local practitioners.

It would be strange indeed if luck alone explained such a concordance of positive results. The success can be attributed to the method. It really is a method that we are talking about here and I have frequently been able to make the following fundamental observation, which I consider to be definitive proof of my assertions. Lausanne is appropriately considered as the Mecca of homoeopathy in my country. For over a century reputed doctors have practised this speciality here and given the city an international reputation that is maintained today by the diversity of skills on offer at our two private schools. There are presently 15 homoeopathic practices in and around the city. On a Swiss scale this is a record. It is therefore possible to speak in terms of competition. This implies a certain freedom for the patients and a welcome possibility for interchange in the event of disagreement. Naturally it has occasionally happened that a patient preferred another doctor's services to mine, and in turn I have often taken on a treatment that had been started by some other homoeopathic colleague. In this way I built up over time a 'repertory' of 15 other methods of practice.

I won't spend any time on the classical practitioners, strict unicists, whose methods are well known to adepts of homoeopathy and are the subject of many widely available publications. This type of practice doesn't interest us in the sense that its possibilities are too often limited by the obstacle of a blocked flow of vital energy. We will instead look at the work of Voll's followers who know, or should know, how to improve reactional capabilities through the judicious use of nosodes. But the patients that I occasionally see from my six or seven Vollian colleagues clearly show that the ohmmetric technique is inadequate in finding the important events of the past and can even be misleading in the hands of a naive practitioner. Here, unfortunately, I must speak out against the teaching of my initial teacher. Almost all the ex-Vollian patients that I see are in a terrible state of energetic imbalance. The Yin–Yang disorder is obvious when the Chinese pulses are checked using Voll's technique. This contrasts markedly with my own patients, who very rapidly recover the lost balance. Why such a difference? The answer is simple: because these unfortunate people didn't receive the corrective nosodes in the sequential order required by Hering's Law and because certain key events had not been detected.

What is the cause of this deficiency? I attribute it to the trap of a facile predispositional diagnosis, that favourite theme of homoeopathic teaching. It is easy for a beginner to identify rapidly the most marked predisposition. It is considerably harder and less glorious to sift the patient's past conscientiously in search of a destabilizing event. This takes time and patience, intelligence and sensitivity. If the doctor fails in this search, the imbalance discovered with the ohmmeter is incorrectly attributed to a weakness of the most visible of the four constitutions. These colleagues then speak of 'tuberculinic blockage' or 'psoric blockage', etc, without realizing the absurdity of these labels. (How could the patient have even been born if the vital energy at one of the four spatiotemporal pillars of his genetic code was 'blocked'?)

As a result, the doctor who has been deluded by this flawed reasoning feels authorized to use the great biotherapeutics. In other words he will start working in depth before completing the indispensable preliminary cleaning of the accumulated residues of the patient's life. In doing this he is creating a severe energetic imbroglio because it is not possible to mix the subtle webs of two different space–time increments with impunity. This classic Mikado effect makes everyone lose a lot of time and prevents these young colleagues from taking on any new patients even though they are at the beginning of their careers.

But lost time isn't the most serious inconvenience of these risky activities. By failing to recognize the Law of the Succession of Forces, the homoeopath exposes his patients to a major risk of definitive constitutional destabilization if this limping treatment is pursued for a number of years.

I will try to make myself better understood by using a mechanical example. The four predispositions can be compared to the four wheelnuts that attach each wheel of a car. When you have to change a wheel you would never completely tighten one nut ahead of the others. Everyone knows that all four nuts must be put in place at the same time and gently turned in sequence until they are all correctly tightened. If this method isn't used, the two flat surfaces will not align properly with each other.

A homoeopath puts his patient into a similar situation if, in declaring him tuberculinic, he administers the tuberculinic nosode alone and in increasingly higher doses over the years. I have seen patients like this who had received over 20 or 30 years anywhere from 15 to 20 doses of Tuberculinum LM or CM with no reference to the seasons or for that matter to any predispositional reality, but based on faith in the Law of Similarity or the ohmmetric readings.

Of course the effects were always spectacular, each time increasing the doctor's prestige. I have met people who approach me with the knowing smile of the unconditional homoeopathic enthusiast and joyously announce, 'Well you homoeopaths really are something! I've just taken a Psorinum LM and been sicker than at any time in my life. It really is incredible that your allopathic colleagues continue to deny the efficiency of your treatment!'

What the unfortunate person doesn't realize is that this LM dose given at the wrong season and with no cyclical counterbalance will influence the course of his life, maintaining the chronic illness for ever. He is impressed by the strength of the reaction instead of being surprised that after 30 years of homoeopathic treatment he is bragging about the fact that there is still not enough regained equilibrium to prevent such a reaction. Maybe he will be luckier than the others who regularly 'benefit' from these energetic treatments and whose miserable looks clearly betray the sad failures of our art.

I could cite numerous examples where the major remedies have been prescribed following exactly the Law of Similarities or Voll's technique. Some patients have received Medorrhinum LM or CM 20 times and none of the other three. Others took Psorinum or Luesinum for 20 years without ever seeing Tuberculinum or Medorrhinum. All these 'defectors' who appeared in my consulting rooms had been treated conscientiously, even masterfully, according to the principal law of homoeopathy . . . but they hadn't been cured! Worse, their condition had clearly been aggravated by these classical treatments. What had happened?

As long as the unilateral prescription of the great constitutional remedies doesn't go beyond the medium potencies, the homoeopath doesn't create a major imbalance, particularly if he is satisfied with the results and doesn't intervene too frequently afterwards. But if he uses strengths of LM or greater he creates a predispositional asymmetry which can only be counterbalanced by use of the other three stabilizers. If the same prescription is repeated exclusively all year long, he is behaving like a mechanic forcing a bolt that has been improperly started into its thread. This unfortunate act leads eventually to the creation of a predispositional 'pathogenesia'. (This neologism explains in Greek that a remedy given too frequently ends up creating the problem it was intended to cure.)

As long as the pathogenesia concerns the reactions of an individual who has been chronically intoxicated with an ordinary remedy, his health is not seriously compromised. If the medication is stopped, the equilibrium will quickly return. In fact this is how homoeopaths test their new remedies. But when a doctor affects, by destabilizing it, the very basis of the genetic code through the unilateral use of a major biotherapeutic, the pathogenesia that results (and which can go all the way to a serious depression, anorexia nervosa, diabetic coma or cancer) is much more difficult to correct. Just try to unscrew an old nut and bolt that has been overtightened!

I hope you can now understand that the severity of the biological punishment that occurs when a doctor misuses his ability to correct ancestral conditions is the result of the blatant infringement of a little–known major law of genetic transmission. In fact, it is through the repeated observation of these deplorable disorders that I came to realize the cyclical nature of the predispositions as well as their total domination by a superior dynamic formalism.

What are these four forces of which I claim to define the chronological sequence? I am not sufficiently erudite to attempt an answer to a question that baffles the great physicists of our century. But the intuitive study of the *I Ching* as well as analogical reasoning have convinced me of the intimate relationship between the four forces, the four seasons, the four constitutions and the four directions of space. It is obvious that these forces, which are dynamic by definition, tend to expand. Since they are inseparably linked by their complementary antagonism, they are necessarily cyclic in nature, the only possible expression of their movement.

This rotatory movement can take a clockwise or anticlockwise direction, depending on the direction of the flow of time. Since by nature we are not capable of imagining the anteriority of the future compared with the past, time is perceived by our reasoning as a movement forward from the past to the present. This obligatory direction implies mathematically the univocal rotation of any associated movement, transforming the cyclical merry-go-round of the four forces into a superb ascending spiral. This is the movement made by a nut as it rises along a bolt. If you reverse the rotation it can only descend. The spiralling progression of any dynamic phenomenon is an irrefutable constant of scientific observation. It determines with the same rigour the spin of an electron and the fantastic helix of the galaxies. It is the central enigma of our expanding universe.

Instinctively, all civilizations before ours have sensed the fundamental rotary duality that distinguishes between good and evil. Rotation to the right has always symbolized constructive, ascending progression, while its opposite (in Latin, *sinister*) has always evoked destruction and misery.

This dualism has been represented many times over the centuries by artists and writers, but no symbol has ever been as perfectly evocative as the fascinating turning cross of Mu, which since the beginning of time has offered humanity the freedom of choice: to conform or not conform to the Law. During that happy time before history, man willingly accepted the formidable strength of the four great forces that the wise impetus of the first Will had put into a clockwise rotation. Political forces, sages, priests and doctors conformed to the injunctions of the right spinning cross, the divine *Sauwastika* of the most ancient Sanskrit texts. At that time there was no illness.

But over the centuries this submission to the Law surreptitiously diminished with the materialist progression of individual egotism. To enjoy something one had to own it. To savour properly an acquired situation one had to institutionalize it. To retain a beneficial idea one had to transform it into a dogma. For all civilizations this was the way that the divine rotation to the right lost its impetus and finally became stuck in the static graphics of great symbols. In the West it became definitively fixed in the immobility of the cross.

But there is an irrefutable fact inherent in the nature of our constantly changing world: what doesn't go forward goes backwards. And the inevitable happened. The materialistic insanity of men coupled with the inevitable entropy of non utilized energy led certain madmen to venture an irreparable act: the inversion of the divine movement of the four great forces. The *Sauwastika* turned to the left became the sinister Swastika. The dangerous forces thus released have now reached such a degree of anticlockwise impetus that our children's genetic codes are being impregnated by them.

Our grandparents were affected mostly by psora and tuberculinism, our immediate generation by sycosis and now our children are strongly tainted with luetism. This predisposition is the last in the order of the succession of forces.

The most recent sign of this is the terrifying disease AIDS, which puts the finishing touches to what any homoeopath will recognize at a glance as the full 'luetic' portrait: an amalgam of religious sectarianism, love of money, outlandish dress, leftist intellectual extremism and homosexuality.

What can be done faced with the amplitude of this threatened disaster? How can the runaway big wheel be stopped? The only intelligent answer to these agonizing questions is once again dictated by common sense. It is we human beings who need to change, and urgently!

Doctors of Real Medicine have the potential to do this. They can help us to change by re-establishing the health of the individual, one by one, ridding each of us of our etheric impurities. But how will they go about this laborious task? You now know: by restarting for everyone, through analogical induction, the majestic circular movement of the four great forces in their original clockwise order of succession – this is the highest ambition of Real Medicine.

TWENTY-THREE

Conclusion: Medicine in the age of Aquarius

This recapitulatory chapter offers those readers interested in the medicine of tomorrow a pot pourri of practical information that will, I hope, stimulate the imagination. Its ideal aim is to create in healthy people a new mental attitude, more demanding and beneficial in the event of illness than an unthinking submission to the authority of the men in white.

The first obstacle to be overcome is fear. This serious character flaw is the doctor's major enemy. I know this all too well since I am a terrible worrier myself and can immediately and sympathetically feel the fundamental concern that a patient shows me, unbeknown to himself, when our eyes meet.

But, while it is perfectly natural for someone who is ill to give way to a certain anxiety, the therapist must stand firm and counter this disempowering feeling with his own willpower. He is helped in this by a major advantage not available to the patient. He knows the illness and its changing forms. This knowledge of the enemy, combined with experience, should give the doctor the indispensable assurance required to eradicate fear. I say 'should' since I must unfortunately acknowledge that my colleagues, rather than relieving the anxiety of their patients, contribute heavily to the universal expansion of the existential cowardice that is the scourge of our materialist civilization.

Why are they so little in control of their own anxiety? Because in refusing the energetic concept of health they fail to recognize the real causes of illness. Allopathic doctors make me think of overarmed soldiers trying to do battle in the dark against a faceless and silent enemy. Every once in a while they grab a germ and battle it to the ground at tremendous cost, then the fear returns and they sit back waiting for the next attack. In the art of medicine, as in the art of war, victory goes to the one who takes the initiative. Only those who know their adversary well will attack. From now on so can you and I.

You know that your life is a flow of vital energy. You also know that because all energy is bipolar, health is conditioned by the dynamic balance of this duality. Illness comes from an obstacle to this harmonious vital expansion. This obstacle itself is necessarily energetic since only one energy can deviate another. I've shown you throughout this book how diverse the nature of this troublemaker can be. It is usually extremely complicated owing to the intricacy of successive events, but it is not indecipherable. Why be afraid when it is possible with the anamnesis alone to identify most of the destabilizing events?

We have reviewed the troublemakers that are most directly accessible to the meticulous questioning of an enquiring mind. You were certainly not surprised to find the events that popular wisdom usually blames for all ill-health: vaccinations, chemical pollution, severe childhood illnesses, surgical operations, and other disturbances. These multiple shocks, modulations of space–time, mark the spatiotemporal fabric of our lives with their immaterial signatures. I have given them priority in this book, the objective of which is to demonstrate their complete neutralization by sequential homoeo- and isopathic therapy.

I have also tried to show that the gravity of energetic destabilization never reaches its full extent without the underhand complicity of a weakened genetic code. The simplest way to wind up the worn-out spring came to me through analogical reasoning. I applied the sequential discipline to the correction of the four angular moments of the spiralled DNA code in the clockwise order imposed by the Law. In the severity of certain cases evoked here you have certainly recognized the hereditary background to major illnesses. I sincerely believe that the complete sequential therapy can both correct minor genetic imperfections and efficiently prevent more serious ones if applied to both parents before they have children.

Obviously this work of compensatory regulation – which will be the daily work of the doctors of tomorrow – must be completed by the manual correction of any physically perceptible imbalances. This is the mission of the osteopaths, who will have replaced other less knowledgeable 'manipulators' within the next 20 years. It is customary for me to tell my patients that the long string of my homoeopathic doses comprises only a third of the ingredients that go into the Real Medicine, which alone is capable of re-establishing and guaranteeing health. The hands of the osteopath are an indispensable complement.

The third pillar of our energetic balance is even more modest in appearance and so discreet that its importance – enormous – goes completely unnoticed by official health administrations. Naturally I am referring here to our food, the structural support of our physical and moral well-being. Since doctors are mostly totally incompetent in this area, we are fortunately responsible individually for our nutritional balance.

This therapeutic triptych constitutes the basis of Real Medicine. In some respects it is even its definition.

When you give it a little thought though, isn't it curious that it is precisely these three directions that medical schools all over the Western world avoid exploring. In most civilized nations, at least in my own country, official teachers do everything in their power to prevent the long-awaited spread of the regulatory techniques of vital energy. Is it an accident that homoeopathy is still not accepted in our universities? Why do our schools of manual techniques prepare only timorous and ineffective physiotherapists when osteopathy is so effective? Why must future doctors spend sleepless nights memorizing useless chemical formulas when they don't even know the virtues of black radish or celery?

No, I don't believe a fortuitous 'accident' deprives medical students of this indispensable three-sided knowledge. By maintaining them in ignorance those in power ensure control over a market as lucrative as armaments but much more hypocritical! This profligate, 'moral' palliative medicine is immeasurably more costly than its modest poor relation, which, into the bargain, can deliver lasting cures. One thing it certainly does know how to do, however, is organize its propaganda. While only benefiting a politico-medico-pharmaceutical clique, it makes us believe that we are all beneficiaries. However, it is no longer possible to hide completely the unappetizing background: just like the armament industry, which is nourished by the atrocity of war, palliative medicine feeds itself on chronic illness and slow death. Both businesses prosper from a cleverly maintained discord. Is it the same hand pulling all the strings? I don't know, but common sense tells me that the harmony of a people is in exact proportion to the sum of each individual's harmony.

How can the threat hanging over the health of human beings and nations be avoided? I believe very strongly that it is within our power to fight victoriously against this dual scourge. Most pressing is the need to ensure to everyone that irreplaceable state of grace represented by a perfect energetic harmony, the first and foremost condition of health. When the most precious thing that we possess is threatened it is up to us alone to choose a medicine that heals before it is too late.

Here is a first piece of advice, an essential *Leitmotiv* of the medicine of tomorrow. Eat what the seasons and your own soil provide. Stop laughing at the courageous people who attempt to reform our eating habits. They are right no matter what the lackeys of the food industry may say. The great civilizations of history have always been built on agricultural prosperity and culinary simplicity. With a bowl of rice, a vegetable and a few animal proteins the Chinese have maintained their surprising cultural superiority for centuries. With a daily portion of whole wheat the ancient legionaries accomplished the 'great works' of the Romans, which we still admire today.

Our bodies are made of what we eat. For centuries human beings were satisfied with the products offered by nature. Our organisms became used to certain rhythms and certain suppliers and were patiently built up from the beginning of time by elements in the immediate environment. Why change this wonderful order? Why eat strawberries in winter when wisdom proposes potatoes and lentils? Why import exotic foods at tremendous cost when each season offers us its diversity?

By deriding the laws of nature thanks to modern techniques, we have slowly 'denaturalized' our food. It has mostly become inert. We must not forget that life creates life. If the food isn't alive, health can't be guaranteed, and food loses its vitality as soon as it is preserved. What could be more logical? Life is energy and energy is space–time. Our old friend time is always there at the heart of all biological phenomena. We all know that no one can control him. That is why preservation is never perfect and is always obtained at the detriment of life.

So follow this first piece of advice to the letter and you will already live more harmoniously with nature and the seasons. Eat a lot of fresh fruit and vegetables that are grown locally, and give a privileged place to the rich cereals that ancient traditions tell us should be eaten whole and freshly ground. Bread used to have such a good taste and be so nourishing because the bakers worked hand in hand with the millers. Flour was always fresh and whole; the precious biological constituents weren't eliminated by sifting or diminished by oxidation.

It is encouraging to see the increasing number of families that bake their own bread at home. Certain households have acquired small household grinders so that they can always have fresh flour available. This is not a passing fashion. It is the first step towards an enormous and necessary alimentary reform. Too bad for the huge industrial flourmills. They have become, along with the agrochemical business and the deterioration of the soil, one of the most treacherous hidden causes of the decline of our civilization.

Avoid white flour as much as possible. Even wheat parasites won't have anything to do with it! Refuse white sugar, refined salt, artificial flavourings, overly sweetened drinks and preserves. Don't ever forget that the food industry cannot replace nature. It merely offers us convenience and its vitamin additives can never return vitality to a product.

I personally am too fond of 'good food' to become a vegetarian, but I admit that the historical examples of Roman legionaries, of small but inexhaustible Asiatic warriors and of undernourished but valiant Afghan resistance-fighters have convinced me of the absurdity of our abusive cult of meat. The proteins of whole grain rice and our traditional cereals are more than equivalent to the polypeptides of meat (after all, meat is nothing more than a dead body). The decomposition of long peptide chains increases with the passage of time following slaughter of the animal. The process can be slowed by intense cold and the use of antioxidants, but no one has yet been able to halt time in such a way as to retain vitality.

Unless you plan to imitate the lion's steaming and bloody meals, you should reduce your consumption of meat to three or four times a week, or even less if you are no longer young. You will be surprised by the increased energy that can be obtained so easily. Too bad for the wealthy livestock breeders. Your relative abstinence will force them to abandon their sordid pillage of the Third World's stocks of grain.

Your gesture will also lighten the overburdened budgets of our Western social security and health systems by several million dollars. This is because of a simple anatomical configuration: the human large intestine is much longer than that of other carnivorous animals. The contact between our digestive mucous system and the toxic residues from the decomposition of animal proteins is therefore significantly prolonged. This biological laxity becomes a dangerous stagnation if the diet doesn't contain enough fibrous elements, and can lead to catastrophe. Constipation opens the door to all kinds of illnesses including cancer and terrible mental depression.

Every day you should eat salads, vegetables, apples and other unpeeled fruit, wholemeal bread, bran, whole cereals and other grains. This is the price of health. Too bad for the stomach doctors, the psychiatrists and the radiologists. If you follow this simple advice you will also help to ruin the practices of the cancer doctors.

A healthy diet is the domestic pillar of Real Medicine. You can strengthen it at your own pace over the years by following any of a thousand recipes known to popular 'folklore' – infusions that purge, large glasses of water every morning before eating, Vermont apple vinegar, Swedish elixirs for longevity, vegetable juice cures, reasonable fasting, etc. The wealth of our cultural patrimony in this area is enormous and generally available in the many healthfood centres that have appeared in all our major cities. If you can find a good herbalist or a real homoeopathic pharmacy, go and make yourself known. The enlightened advice of a competent person may help you avoid the risk of having to consult a half-doctor. Always ask for the owner, because this will encourage him to persevere in his choice of following a less lucrative and unselfish path.

If you know of an excellent naturopath or a 'whole' (not half!) doctor, stay with them. They are still few and far between in our world and are worth their weight in gold. If you are not so lucky you will have to be satisfied with a half-diagnosis by your allopath, which can be a little more instructive than the small-talk of a common naturopath. This is what my patients do when they are unable to reach me and want to know immediately the nature of some unexpected problem.

Intelligent people care for themselves with rest (in bed if necessary), plenty of fluids, light foods, vegetable juices, apple vinegar, poultices, enemas and whatever other similar commonsense things may come to mind. Add herbal infusions, oligoelements, essential oils, Chinese massage, acupuncture and household homoeopathy and you have a good assortment of efficient therapies. Why add chemicals? I willingly admit to a weakness for the ferocious logic of the American school of natural medicine, which basically says the following:

> If you're well it would never enter your head to swallow a chemical pill. You would be much too afraid of poisoning yourself. Why then would you consider doing it when you're sick? Is your weakened organism any better able to deal with the intoxication?

This formula delights me because of the deeper truth that it encompasses and I offer it for your meditation before proposing the advice that I really consider to be most important. It concerns fever. Please once and for all stop fearing this gift. Nature isn't stupid. It's not without reason that she has allowed herself such an enormous exception to the sacrosanct principle of thermal stability that is usually so well protected by the proven mechanisms of self-regulation. The high temperatures of a fever prevent the proliferation of germs and it would be a great pity to block this beneficial aid with medication.

Let the natural defences operate. They require only discreet support and suffer from being continuously impeded in their action. With fever, a daily dose of the oligo-element copper advantageously replaces antibiotics and antipyretic drugs. It also stimulates the reticuloendothelial system, that organizer of the counter-attacks to aggression. Copper should be part of all family medicine cabinets. It is far superior to aspirin and is all that is required to put rapidly in place a first line of active defence in our infectious struggles against childhood illness, colds, flus, sore throats, earaches, furunculosis, bacterial rheumatism, meningitis, hepatitis, etc. With the additional help of the major homoeopathic remedies for fever, anyone can easily master an early infection, and occasionally avoid the trouble and expense of a doctor.

And what are the names of these precious aides? The most famous are called Aconitum, Belladonna, Ferrum phosphoricum, Eupatorium perfoliatum and Gelsemium. These five stars should under no circumstances be missing from your medicine cabinet. I won't describe their characteristics here since you can find this information in any general book on homoeopathy. Memorize them all, but retain Belladonna in particular. It is unsurpassed at the beginning of any childhood illness that it allows to express itself in a natural way. If a fever goes above 40°C (104°F) you shouldn't hesitate to give a dose of Belladonna 9C, MK or even XMK. In doing so you will remove the threat of delirium, that terror of young mothers and doctors blinded by fear of possible cerebral effects. But remember one thing. By administering this king of remedies you will not achieve a sudden drop in the temperature. As I said earlier, that is not the goal. You are merely directing the defensive energies in the proper direction. That is enough. I have been doing this for the last 9 years. Even frightening scarlet fever itself can be defused in this manner without antibiotic masquerade and without complications.

And since I'm giving advice, here is some that is so practical that it will make all the trouble you've taken to read this book worthwhile. Go out right away and buy yourself several doses of Arnica in potencies of 5, 7 and 9C. This friendly mountain plant is absolutely miraculous in any kind of traumatism, provided it is absorbed in its homoeopathic form and not just applied externally as a liquid or ointment. Arnica cannot replace surgery, but it can transform the prognosis for torn ligaments and broken bones and greatly shorten the recovery period. In 5 and 7C it is sufficient to overcome the pain of small wounds and the swelling of bruises. In 9C it can save a crushed nail or cure a sprain. In the case of severe mental or physical shock, it is absolutely indispensable to give at least a 9 or 12C immediately. This simple act can modify the destiny of its recipient.

Arnica should have a place in all sport bags, in all first-aid kits, in the pockets of your ski outfit, in bicycle bags, cars, homes, schools, in fact everywhere. Of all remedies, Arnica is the one that is most immediately beneficial provided the recipient is receptive to homoeopathy. In this respect it is doubly precious since it serves as a test. If the positive effects are immediate then the person has a good reactional capability. If this is not the case then the person should probably immediately start a cure of sequential cleaning.

I would also like to correct the widespread opinion that homoeopathy is beneficial only to the young and becomes totally inefficient with age. I have indirectly and involuntarily contributed to the spread of this idea myself since I generally won't accept any older patients in order to give priority to children. This choice is not a discriminatory whim. The explanation is tragically simple. When a boat is sinking, the first places in the lifeboats are reserved for children and their mothers. Unfortunately the menace to public health has never been as great as today at the close of this materialist civilization. The human species has never before run such a risk of definitive genetic destabilization. The great plagues of history didn't kill all reproductive ability, but mutant overvaccination and antibiotic madness spare no one.

Given the imminence of the irreversible catastrophe that threatens our genetic integrity, I have tried over the years to save one or two children each day from the degrading control of modern paediatrics. This is the main reason that gave me the energy to overcome my horror of writing, and I would be more than pleased if critics consider my book for what it really is: a strident alarm bell.

Yes, I hope that I have been able to make you see that the medicine of tomorrow won't be prepared in the laboratories of the pharmaceutical industry, but rather in the complete remodelling of our scientific dogma. The main theme of this cultural revolution is prevention. It is not after having mistreated his energetic balance for years that a patient should put himself in someone else's hands and simply pay the bill for his thoughtlessness. Through recognition of the different space–time increments that come together to form life, an intelligent person gives himself the means to track down at an early stage any slight alteration in any of them. If dietary energy is the cause, it can be immediately and easily corrected since it is often only the result of laziness or habit.

If the confusion is mechanical, the patient can call a mechanic to correct rapidly that wonderful ingredient of vital energy that can be felt with the hands. The medicine of tomorrow will use osteopathy extensively and will place it at the head of all manual techniques. In the America of the 1930s, Edgar Cayce was really an outsider in his frequent prescriptions of osteopathic corrections. Today in the same country the professional association of these new doctors is as powerful as that of the others. Osteopaths no longer allow themselves to be intimidated by allopathic pseudoscientific pedantry. They have the approval of a public that is pleased with their economical efficiency.

The day when intelligent obstetricians and midwives demand the presence of an osteopath at their sides in the delivery rooms, civilization will take a huge step forward. It is impossible to measure the positive impact that immediate correction, with bare hands, has on the inevitable cranial deformations at birth. This simple gesture of remodelling the skull, once practised by the Celts, can prevent numerous problems of behaviour, vision, hearing, mastication, cardiac and respiratory functions, etc in adulthood. Ideally there would be a return to the squatting position for delivery, which was so unfortunately abandoned in the 17th century owing to the combined effects of academic dogmatism and the immeasurable human capacity for stupidity. Certain pioneers like Dr Paciornik in Curitiba, Brazil, and Dr Michel Odent, originally in France and now in England, are already devoting themselves to this cause. It is urgent that we imitate them.

I sincerely believe that the young women of today who are active in sports and physical exercise would be very pleased to accept the partial demedicalization of pregnancy and its final act. They would be ready to approach those 9 months of double life with the same attitude that any athlete has to a physical activity, one of concern for proper preparation and condition. A natural delivery has to be prepared. It requires good physical condition – flexibility, free movement of the pelvic joints and the backbone. Here again osteopathy is queen, particularly if the therapist adds truly corrective gymnastics (like the wonderful method of Mlle Mézières).

Naturally, narrow-minded obstetricians will oppose with all their might this rehabilitation of nature in the delivery room. Dr Paciornik claims a 91 per cent rate of normal deliveries (ie without forceps or scalpel) in 4,000 pregnancies of educated European women brought to a successful conclusion with his methods. You can well imagine the financial ruin that this triumph of common sense implies for those virtuosos of the scalpel that our modern birth attendants have become. Public health and its budgets will be all the better off for it.

But, while waiting for the arrival of intelligence in the teaching of obstetrics, I advise future mothers getting ready to confront the inevitable series of incorrect steps of our current practitioners to enrol the help of a good osteopath. This practitioner is master of the only thing that Real Medicine can usefully oppose to the enormous and unsuspected damage caused by induced births, axis traction, vacuum extractors, forceps and Caesarean delivery. (Induced birth removes the child from the initiative of the natural onset of labour, breaking the harmony between the two vital energies which are then brutally thrown out of phase. The primary cranial breathing of the child is incorrectly modulated and seriously disturbed by the artificial violence of the uterine contractions. The traction on the head has the same effects to a lesser degree, and vacuum extractors and forceps are the same but worse. As for Caesarean birth, it bypasses the beneficial and rhythmically timed cranial modelling of nature whose determining subtleties we are only beginning to imagine.)

From the outset, pregnancy is the privileged moment for prevention. I am not speaking here of the programmes of prenatal eugenics that certain schools of homoeopathy propose to the public. The use of the major constitutional biotherapeutics without seasonal references and a preliminary isopathic and sequential cleaning seems to me to be ill-conceived. It can cause very spectacular imbalances, which I have had occasion to see in certain French children who had received this hazardous preventive treatment. In my opinion the only eugenics deserving of the name is practised before conception and obtained by applying the complete sequential therapy to both of the future parents.

After fertilization has occurred, medicine's role diminishes in favour of personal initiative. Dietetics become the unquestionable leader of the preventive operations. If the young mother wants to bring a perfectly healthy baby into the world all she has to do is follow Dr Kousmine's instructions and eat a Budwig cream every morning (*see* the Glossary for the recipe). Alternatively, if the young woman eats less nutritional food, all that is required is a dietary supplement in the form of oligo-elements (manganese–copper twice a week and fluor once a week) and attention to fibre intake in order to avoid constipation. I personally never give synthetic vitamins during a pregnancy and almost never give iron. In case of anaemia, the manganese–copper is usually enough to re-establish the level that is indispensable to life.

Children who come into families that are hostile to chemistry are generally superb babies, robust, calm and happy. If the osteopath can repair the mistreatment inflicted by the gynaecologist/obstetrician, the child will rapidly enjoy remarkable health that will surprise other mothers who are still under the influence of the allopaths. The baby's first fevers are related to teething and can be handled without the paediatrician by using increasing doses of Chamomilla in 5, 7 or 9C. Along with the oligoelement copper, Belladonna and Arnica, this other great childhood remedy completes the minimal assortment you need in your home medicine cabinet.

The child grows older, and if vaccinated at 8 or 10 months using the technique described in Chapter 11, his vital energy won't be destabilized and his health will remain excellent. Occasional breaks in harmony that are created by the inevitable childhood illnesses are not very consequential if the morbid shock wave is aided in its expansion by Belladonna and its other homoeopathic helpers. A high potency of the nosode 3 weeks after the start of the illness is all that's needed to remove the final spatiotemporal distortions that have been created by the virulence of the event.

This is how the medicine of tomorrow should be understood. Its therapeutic effect must instantaneously grasp the here and now. By accompanying nature in its regulatory effort, the doctor prevents a residual destabilization of the vital energy. The patient loses his balance only for a brief moment then quickly recovers. You will understand that, in so doing, medicine progressively loses its therapeutic vocation and accedes to the more noble rank of health guardian.

For patients returned to health by sequential therapy the subsequent objective of Real Medicine is limited to the erasures as they occur of the smallest sequels left by the shocks of life. The lucky babies who have the advantage of this intelligent surveillance starting from their arrival in this world are obviously very privileged. Tomorrow they will be the people of Aquarius. But the other children – and everyone who is ill – must not be neglected. I sincerely hope that they will all one day meet a real doctor who will take control of their destinies. If that colleague finds inspiration in these pages I will not have worked in vain.

It is obvious that sequential therapy is not the cure-all that suffering humanity so anxiously awaits. I am fully aware of its limits. But if the method isn't perfect, it can be perfected. Study of my failures has led me to make certain surprising discoveries, which comfort me in the thought that the homoeopathic simillimum absolutely must be improved in order to become the true isopathic simile. This effort is the price of perfection.

My current preoccupations involve allergy research. I can cure eight hayfever cases out of ten using the triple combination that I have described. But why should I have to put up with the disappointment of failure in the other two cases? An amusing story about insects gave me a hint. Here it is.

My mother was one of the first experimental volunteers of my sequential therapy. It did her a great deal of good but I had been unable to rid her of certain allergic symptoms uncommon for her age. At a certain point I remembered that her legs had once been very badly bitten by an army of bedbugs that had taken up residence in the cane seats of a cinema in Indochina. I was taken with a fanciful idea (and encouraged by a secret hope) and sent her a highly potentized dose of Cimex (Latin for bedbug). The result was instantaneous. She called me the next day to say that for a few hours her legs had swelled and once again looked like the tree trunks that had so frightened her a half century earlier. Ever since that fantastic isopathic revival her allergic tendencies have significantly diminished.

This extraordinary experience proves that the smallest events in our lives can interfere with the delicate mechanisms of our most sophisticated regulatory systems and play the role of the grain of sand that can cause the whole machine to break down.

This adventure taught me that the correct sequence is the hardest thing to find, even with the ever-so-precious help of radiesthesia. It may seem impossible to capture all the little accidents of a lifetime, but allergological experiments have shown that it is mostly injected substances, which are foreign to human beings, that have the greatest destabilizing powers.

Beware of the common Mantoux tuberculin test, or any kind of intradermal skin tests and of injections of animal or vegetal albuminoid substances. Be aware that many vaccines are prepared using animal-based biological supports. Their use must be urgently abandoned in favour of vaccines prepared from human serums. You should also be aware that the innumerable new chemically synthesized molecules are not particularly well-liked by our organisms, which haven't learned to live with them as they did over millions of years with the molecules invented by nature.

No one can say exactly what occurs with a 'toximolecular' remedy that is imposed by force through the natural barrier of the skin. This violent intrusion can only create disorder and problems. Knowing that nature always takes its revenge, even for minor violations, it's hard not to shudder thinking of the consequences threatening patients who have received frequent injections. I read in the very serious *Journal of the American Medical Association* that the sperm of young US Army soldiers contains DDT, and that one can see in this a plausible explanation for the worrisome current progression of male sterility. What sin have these young men committed? All they did was eat the products of a chemically dependent agricultural system. How then will we end up paying for everything that we absorb in considerably less natural ways?

The medicine of tomorrow will carefully avoid injections of artificial drugs. Don't smile in disbelief; this isn't a prophecy. Thousands of patients treated with biocompatible methods have already forgotten the poignant memories of medical injections. You need only do the same by refusing allopathy's poisoned favours. If you don't have the courage yourselves to throw away these chemical crutches then at least you should have the intelligence to spare your children this completely unjustified violence.

For pity's sake, protect them! Children are far more vulnerable than we are. Simple common sense tells us that their organisms aren't yet fully formed. Biology teaches us that their defensive systems are immature because temporarily lacking the complex neuroendocrine organization. The younger the child the greater is the risk of permanent distortion to a marvellous equilibrium. Irreversible lesions are almost certain when interventions take place a few hours following birth. So-called 'wild' animals know this instinctively and protect their offspring to the death.

The medicine of tomorrow cannot be built on the misery of innocents. It doesn't require animal sacrifices and couldn't care less about costly teams of researchers drunk with images of pseudoscientific glory. This new medicine is being prepared thoughtfully and in observance of nature. It is an intellectual exercise that is open to everyone and in which we can all participate, submitting our theoretical visions to the difficult confrontation with reality. Often a person who seeks honestly will have to modify his initial concepts in order to progress little by little towards truth. He knows that patience doesn't dishonour this activity, which will ultimately bring science and conscience together.

I know that my E cycle isn't perfect. Repeated failure with patients of strong allergic hereditary backgrounds has dictated certain useful therapeutic variations. I now more frequently use certain types of homoeopathic tuberculins improperly considered rare. A naturopath friend also reminded me of the impact on our genetic codes of the plague epidemics of the past. This brilliant idea is not just an intellectual construction. Yersin's nosode (the Swiss Alexander Yersin discovered the plague bacillus in 1894) can sometimes bring about a spectacular recovery if incorporated at the right place in the EI or EII cycle.

For my part I think I have found the principal flaw in the E cycle: the kind of tuberculinic nosodes being used. I may make this discovery the subject of a later publication if future practice confirms the accuracy of my theory. I also still have to try to put together a major classification of the inductors and drainers according to their predispositional families and their strange biophysical properties.

It is not work that is lacking for the pioneers of this medicine which heals. Although it may seem enormous, the effort required is not superhuman. It must first take place in the mind as a matter of urgent priority before it can take on a more concrete form in the laboratories.

In fact it is really only a change of direction. When the researchers of the entire world have realized that biochemistry is merely a vassal to particle physics, then medicine will at last be able to strike out on the royal road.

Glossary

Aetiology

The causes of diseases.

Allopathy

A term widely used to describe orthodox medicine. It was coined by Hahnemann to differentiate it from the method he had discovered. Orthodox medicine uses agents that have a contrary effect to the pathology in question – eg a fever is treated by an anti-inflammatory agent. The term comes from the Greek *allos* meaning 'other', hence allopathic. Doctors practising this method are called 'allopaths'. The Greek for 'similar' is *homoion*, hence homoeopathy – like causes like.

Anamnesis

Recollection of all the pathological conditions and their treatments that have taken place in the subject's life, established in chronological order.

Anthroposophic medicine

System of medicine based on the harmonization of the physical and spiritual sides of human beings, introduced by Rudolph Steiner (1861–1925), an Austrian scholar, mystic and teacher.

Astral body

Our 'third' body. The immaterial organism at the basis of our emotional life.

BCG

An antituberculosis vaccination compulsory in France.

Biotherapeutic

Homoeopathic remedies prepared from pathological or non-pathological secretions or excretions of non-chemically defined microbic substances, having their source in animal or plant tissues.

Budwig cream

Dr C Kousmine named her famous recipe after the German pharmacist who suggested the first elements to her.

Per person:

- 2 tsp good quality linseed oil (cold-pressed)
- 4 tsp of fat-free cream cheese or yoghurt.

  Whip the oil and the cream cheese into a smooth cream, then add:
- the juice of half a lemon
- one mashed ripe banana, or 2 tsp of honey
- one grated apple, or fruit of the season
- 2 tsp of raw wholegrain cereals, freshly ground (the choice is yours: wheat, buckwheat, oats, millet, whole rice, etc, but never mix the cereals)
- 2 tsp of various oleaginous seeds (linseed, sunflower, sesame, almonds, etc).

C

One of two different types of dynamizations or potencies. (See K for the other.) C for centesimal consists of successive successed dilutions of one part of the original substance combined with 99 parts of a soluble excipient, changing each time into a different bottle (called a Hahnemannian dilution). The first succussion is called 1C (often written just as 1). One 100th part of this is transferred to a second bottle with 99 parts of soluble excipient and the process is repeated to give 2C, and so on.

(Normally, in the English-speaking world, potencies are in centesimal unless stated otherwise. For instance, Nux vomica 30 is Nux vomica 30C.)

DTPP

A combined vaccination against diphtheria, tetanus, whooping cough and polio, also known as DiTePerPol.

Endogenic

A process that has its cause within the organism itself.

Etheric body

Our 'second' body. The immaterial organism at the basis of the life of our physical body.

Homoeopathy

Therapy invented by Samuel Hahnemann, a German doctor who was born in Saxony in 1755 and died in Paris in 1843. It is based on the principle (already known to Hippocrates) that like cures like. The genius of Hahnemann was to discover that a substance producing a particular pattern of symptoms in a healthy individual would cure an illness producing the same pattern of symptoms if administered in infinitesimal doses (dilutions or potencies) 'dynamized' or 'potentized' by succussions. The individual person's reaction to the disease is treated rather than the disease itself.

Iatrogenic

Toxic effect produced by allopathic remedies themselves.

Isotherapeutic

A homoeopathic remedy obtained from the substance that has caused the health problems.

K or Korsakovian

A method of preparing dilutions invented by General Korsakov, a Russian who was physician to the Czar. The principle is the same as for centesimal except that a single bottle is used. Korsakov estimated that when the bottle was emptied after the first succussion approximately 100th part remained on the inner surface of the bottle and that it was thus unnecessary to change the bottle each time.

MMR

A combined vaccination against mumps, measles and German measles (rubella).

Neurasthenic

A person suffering from neurasthenia, a pathological condition characterized by nervous depression and various physical manifestations.

Nosode

A homoeopathic remedy obtained from the germ or virus that has caused the illness.

Oligo-elements

Catalytic trace elements. The oligo-elements referred to in this book are available from French pharmacies, with the major brand (Labcatal) selling them under the name of Oligosols. The range includes metals (aluminium, copper, magnesium, etc) and minerals (sulphur, phosphorous, etc).

Radiesthesia

The use of a pendulum for diagnostic and prescribing purposes.

Sedimentation rate

A biological test that measures the rate at which red blood cells are deposited in a test-tube. It indicates certain pathological states, notably inflammatory ones.

Serocytol therapy

Treatment by biological serums specific to the organ or tissue of which the immunity is to be reinforced.

Simillimum

The unique remedy that corresponds exactly to the pathology of the patient.

Select bibliography

(The bulk of this appendix has been voluntarily reduced to a few titles of which the contents express clearly one or another leading idea of this present book.)

Chapter 1

H-Ch Geffroy, *Tu vivras cent ans*, CEVIC Editeur, 94520 Mandres Les Roses 1978 (the philosophy of the founder of La Vie Claire).

Dr Jacques Ménétrier, *La médecine des fonctions.* Le François, Paris 1974 (biological catalysis).

Dr Victor Pauchet, *Le chemin du bonheur. La rééducation de soi-même*, Editions J Oliven, Paris 1929 (dietetics and hygiene).

Dr Victor Pauchet, *Restez jeunes*, Editions J Oliven, Paris 1931.

Dr A De Sambucy, *Les deux sources de la médecine européene.* Dangles, Paris 1968 (the importance of the spinal column).

Chapter 3

Samuel Hahnemann, *Doctrine homéopathique ou Organon de l'Art de guérir*, translated from the sixth German edition, Librairie Jeheber, Geneva 1975.

Samuel Hahnemann *Organon of Medicine*, 1810; New translation by Kunzli, Naude and Pendleton, Tarcher, Los Angeles 1982.

Chapter 4

Dr Reinhold Voll, *Medikamententestung, Nosodentherapie und Mesenchymreaktivierung*, ML-Verlag, Uelzen 1976.

Chapter 7

Fritjof Capra, *Le Tao de la physique*, Tchou, Paris 1979. (English edition: *The Tao of Physics*, Bantam, New York 1977.)

Fritjof Capra, *Le temps du changement*, Editions du Rocher, Monaco 1983.

(English edition: *The Turning Point,* Bantam, New York 1982.)
Jean E Charon, *L'esprit, cet inconnu,* Albin Michel, Paris 1977.
Jean E Charon, *Mort, voici ta défaite,* Albin Michel, Paris 1979 (the qualities of the electron).

Chapter 8

Etienne Guillé, *L'alchimie de la vie,* Editions du Rocher, Monaco 1984 (radiesthesia and mathematics).
Sheila Ostrander and Lynn Schroeder, *Psychic Discoveries Behind the Iron Curtain.*
Charles Terreaux, *Maîtrisez votre santé,* Editions P-M Favre, Lausanne 1982 (the physical parameters of health, revealed to medical doctors by a physicist).

Chapter 13

Dr Paul Chavanon, *La guerre microbienne est commencée* (Bacterial War Has Started), Dangles, Paris 1950 (the imposture of BCG).
Simone Delarue, *Les vaccinations dans la vie quotidienne.*
Dr Ferru, *La faillite du BCG,* Ligue Nationale pour la Liberté des Vaccinations, 4, rue Saulnier, Paris 9e 1978.
Edmond Székely, *L'Evangile de la Paix de Jésus-Christ par le disciple Jean,* P Genillard Editeur, Lausanne (teachings of Jesus on dietetics and hygiene).

Chapter 16

Dr Jean Gauthier, *L'enfant, ce glandulaire inconnu,* Albi 1961 (the physical bases of mental illness).
Jacqueline Gauthey-Urwyler, *Manger sainement pour bien se porter,* Delachaux & Niestlé, Neuchâtel-Paris 1984.
Dr Catherine Kousmine, *Soyez bien dans votre assiette jusqu' à 80 ans et Plus,* Tchou, Paris 1980.
Dr Catherine Kousmine, *La sclérose en plaques est guérissable,* Delachaux & Niestlé, Neuchâtel 1984.
Carl C Pfeiffer and Pierre Gonthier, *Equilibre psycho-biologique et oligo-eliments,* Debard, Paris 1983.
Dr Anthony J Sattilaro, *Rappelé à la vie,* Calman-Lévy, Paris 1983 (the treatment of cancer by macrobiotics).

Chapter 17

Lionelle Issartel and Marielle Issartel, *L'ostéopathie exactement,* Editions Laffont, Paris 1983.

Chapter 22

Louis-Claude Vincent, *Le paradis perdu de MU,* Editions la Source d'Or, Marsat 1975 (Sauwastika and Swastika).

Chapter 23

Dr D C Jarvis, *Ces vieux remèdes qui guérissent,* Laffont, Paris 1962 (vinegar and cider and health). (English edition: *Folk Remedies for Healing.*)

Dr Paciornik, *Apprenez l'accouchement accroupi!* Editions P-M Favre, Lausanne 1982.

Index